D1145317

COLOUR GUIDE

Infectious Diseases

Peter Ball FRCPEd
Honorary Senior Lecturer
School of Biomedical Sciences
University of St. Andrews
St. Andrews
Scotland

James A. Gray FRCPEd
Formerly Consultant Infectious Disease Physician
City Hospital
Edinburgh
Scotland

SECOND EDITION

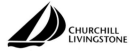
CHURCHILL
LIVINGSTONE

EDINBURGH LONDON MADRID MELBOURNE NEW YORK
SAN FRANCISCO TOKYO 1998

CHURCHILL LIVINGSTONE
Division of Harcourt Brace & Co Ltd

First published as Colour Aids Infectious Diseases
1984
First Colour Guide edition 1993
Second Colour Guide edition 1998

ISBN 0 443 0 57710 ✓

British Library Cataloguing in Publication Data
A catalogue record for this book is available from
the British Library.

**Library of Congress Cataloging in Publication
Data**
A catalog record for this book is available from
the Library of Congress.

Medical knowledge is constantly
changing. As new information
becomes available, changes in
treatment, procedures, equipment
and the use of drugs become
necessary. The editors/authors/
contributors and the publishers
have, as far as it is possible,
taken care to ensure that the
information given in this text is
accurate and up to date.
However, readers are strongly
advised to confirm that the
information, especially with
regard to drug usage, complies
with current legislation and
standards of practice.

Produced by Addison
Wesley Longman China
Limited, Hong Kong
SWTC/01

The
publisher's
policy is to use
**paper manufactured
from sustainable forests**

For Churchill Livingstone

Publisher: Timothy Horne
Project Editor: James Dale
Production: Nancy Arnott
Design direction: Erik Bigland

Acknowledgements

The authors gratefully acknowledge the kind permission of the following colleagues and others to reproduce photographs from their collections: Dr P. Buxton (Figs 16, 17), Dr B. Dhillon (Figs 39, 61, 163), the late Dr E. Edmond (Fig. 12), Dr D. Felix (Figs 164, 165, 167), Dr R. Hume (Figs 35, 59, 60, 62), Dr J. Innes (Fig. 129), Dr D. H. Kennedy (Fig. 40), Dr C. L. S. Leen (Figs 168, 169), Dr M. McDonald (Figs 57, 58), Dr A. Scott (Fig. 101), Dr B. Watt (Fig. 68), Dr P. D. Welsby (Fig. 42) and Abbot Laboratories Ltd. (Figs 85, 86).

Special thanks are due to the Medical Photography Department, Victoria Hospital, Kirkcaldy, Fife.

Note: Treatment recommendations are general indications only and the reader must consult current prescribing data with regard to dosage (especially in children) and compliance with legislation and standards of practice before treatment of individual patients.

Contents

Measles

Aetiology

Measles virus, a single serotype paramyxovirus.

Incidence

Previously common in preschool and junior schoolchildren, notably in the last few months of the year, the disease is now rare due to widespread effective immunization. Where present, measles is now usually sporadic or sub-epidemic. Explosive outbreaks may occur if measles is introduced to unexposed and non-immune communities.

Pathogenesis

Case to case spread follows airborne droplet transmission from the respiratory tract of patients with active measles. There is no other reservoir of infection. Invasion of the upper respiratory tract and conjunctivae is followed by multiplication in lymphoid tissues and viraemia. Histological appearances are characterized by a mononuclear reaction with giant cells and endothelial proliferation. Lesions are present in skin (rash), mucous membranes (Koplik's spots), lungs, gut and lymphoid tissue.

Clinical features

The incubation period of 2 weeks is followed by the prodromal phase, characterized by upper respiratory catarrh with Koplik's spots on the buccal mucosa (Fig. 1), accompanied by conjunctivitis, otitis media and rhinitis (Fig. 2). 24–48h later a dusky red maculopapular rash commences on the face and spreads peripherally via the trunk (Fig. 3, Fig. 4, p. 4). Uncomplicated measles lasts for 7–10 days, following which the fading rash leaves skin staining (see Fig. 5, p. 4), brown macules with fine desquamation, which can persist for up to 3 weeks.

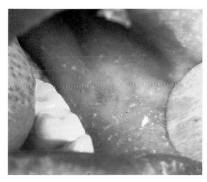

Fig. 1 Koplik's spots on buccal mucosa.

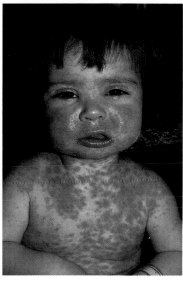

Fig. 2 Morbilliform rash, conjunctivitis and rhinitis.

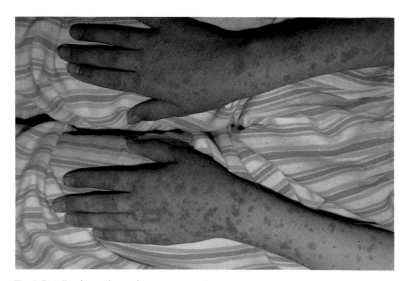

Fig. 3 Details of measles rash.

Complications	• Secondary bacterial *otitis media, bronchopneumonia* and *purulent conjunctivitis*: caused by pneumococci, *Haemophilus influenzae*, less commonly *Staphylococcus aureus*. • *Obstructive laryngitis and dysentery*: associated with childhood and infant malnutrition in developing countries. • *Appendicitis*: increased incidence in measles. • *Giant cell pneumonitis*: a rare diffuse pulmonary infiltration causing respiratory failure. • *Allergic encephalomyelitis* (Fig. 6): onset 1–2 weeks after measles. Incidence 1 : 6000 cases. • *Subacute sclerosing panencephalitis*: reactivation of latent virus within brain after 5–7 years causing encephalitis, fatal within 6–12 months. Incidence 1 : 1 000 000 cases. • *Atypical measles*: hyperpyrexia, vesicular rash and pneumonia. Historically seen in adults hypersensitized by inactivated vaccines used in the 1960s.
Treatment	Management is largely symptomatic. Macrolides, e.g. erythromycin, clarithromycin or azithromycin, or co-amoxiclav are effective for bacterial complications. There is no effective antiviral therapy for acute complications such as pneumonitis. Steroids are of marginal value in allergic encephalitis. Isoprinosine may temporarily arrest progression of sclerosing panencephalitis but does not affect eventual fatal outcome.
Prevention	Notifiable in the UK: hospitalized cases must be isolated. 1. *Active immunization*: attenuated vaccine gives 97% seroconversion and long-term immunity. Mild febrile reactions occur in 3% of vaccinees. In the UK universal immunization, using combined measles/mumps/rubella (MMR) vaccine, is given between 12–18 months of age. The disease has become rare as a result. 2. *Passive immunization*: human normal immunoglobulin protects if given within 72 h of exposure. This is useful in immunocompromised non-immune children.

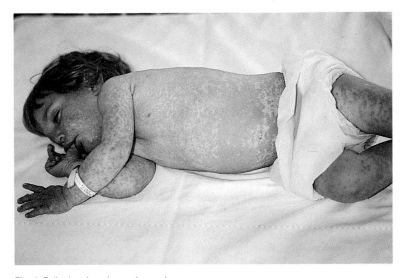

Fig. 4 Fully developed measles rash.

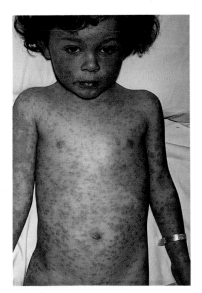

Fig. 5 Post-measles staining.

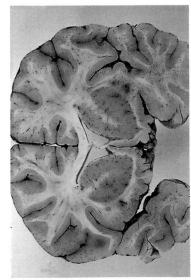

Fig. 6 Measles encephalitis: macropathology.

Rubella

Aetiology | Rubella virus, a single serotype togavirus.

Incidence | Previously observed in schoolchildren with occasional epidemic fluctuations but now rare in immunized western populations.

Pathogenesis | Case-to-case airborne droplet transmission from the respiratory tract of active cases. Invasion by the upper respiratory tract is followed by dissemination to skin, conjunctivae and mucous membranes and a resultant mild mononuclear reaction and proliferative hyperplasia in lymph nodes. Lesions occur in the skin, lymphoid tissue, conjunctivae.

Clinical features | The incubation period of 2.5–3 weeks is followed by mild upper respiratory catarrh, conjunctival suffusion and, within 24–48 h, a discrete maculopapular generalized rash (Figs 7–10). In contrast to measles, Koplik's spots are not seen and systemic upset and irritability are minimal. Lymphadenopathy is prominent, notably of suboccipital and post-auricular groups. The rash may last 5 days but is often fleeting and fades without staining or desquamation. Rubella is diagnosed by the haemagglutination-inhibition and IgM tests.

Complications |
- *Immune complex arthritis*: transient, non-deforming and typically affecting small joints. Incidence 10%—mainly in women.
- *Allergic encephalomyelitis*: commences 10–14 days after rubella. Incidence 1 : 6000.
- *Purpura*: caused by thrombocytopenia and vascular defects (rare).
- *Congenital rubella syndrome* (p. 7).

Treatment | Management is symptomatic. Non-steroidal anti-inflammatory agents may be required for rubella arthritis.

Prevention | Not notifiable in the UK: hospitalized cases must be isolated. Live attenuated rubella vaccines (Cendehill and RA27/3 strains) give high level protection. In the UK immunization is accomplished using combined measles/mumps/rubella (MMR) vaccine given between 12–18 months of age.

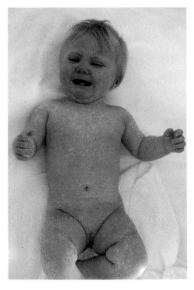

Fig. 7 Infantile rubella rash.

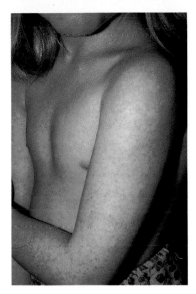

Fig. 8 Discrete macular rash.

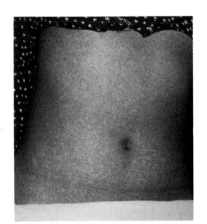

Fig. 9 Profuse rash in adult.

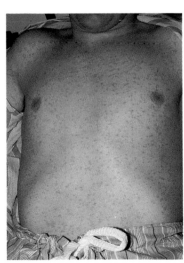

Fig. 10 Sparse rubella rash in adult.

Congenital rubella syndrome (CRS)

Aetiology

Rubella virus (p. 5).

Incidence

Affects up to 40% of fetuses exposed to maternal rubella during first trimester. Prior to the present MMR immunization of both sexes, about 60 cases per year occurred in the UK despite the adolescent female prevention programme.

Pathogenesis

Follows transplacental fetal infection by rubella virus. Highest risk between 6–8 weeks' gestation but possible risk up to 16–18 weeks. Widespread fetal involvement includes persistent infection of liver, heart, CNS, lungs, pancreas and long bones. Neonatal jaundice and purpura are often present. Dysorganogenesis results in major ophthalmic, cardiac, auditory and neurological abnormalities in 10% of affected pregnancies.

Clinical features

Severe CRS may include: pulmonary stenosis, persistent ductus arteriosus (common), coarction and ventricular septal defect (rare) (Fig. 11); microphthalmia, cataract (Fig. 12) and retinitis; sensorineural deafness and microcephaly. Severe mental deficiency is uncommon. The extended syndrome may include purpura, anaemia, metaphyseal dysplasia, hepatitis, myocarditis, pneumonitis and low birth weight.

Treatment

Non-immune mothers who develop clinical or serological evidence of rubella in early pregnancy ($<$15 weeks) are offered therapeutic abortion. Rubella immune globulin does not prevent congenital rubella.

Prevention

In the UK immunization is accomplished using combined measles/mumps/rubella (MMR) vaccine given between 12–18 months of age. Non-immune pregnant women exposed to rubella who do not seroconvert must be immunized in the immediate puerperium. The live attenuated (RA 27/3 and Cendehill strain) vaccines available for this purpose must never be administered during pregnancy.

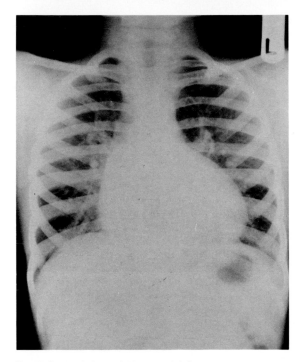

Fig. 11 Congenital ventricular septal defect.

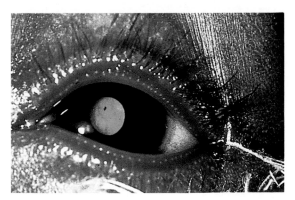

Fig. 12 Congenital rubella cataract.

Mumps

Aetiology	Mumps virus, a single serotype paramyxovirus.
Incidence	All ages may be affected; more common in children over 1 year. Subclinical infection is common. World-wide distribution before widespread availability of effective live attenuated vaccine. Previously 4-year cycles, clustering in spring and winter.
Pathogenesis	Moderately infectious: spreads by airborne droplet transmission from active cases. This is followed by viraemia and glandular involvement. Salivary glands: interstitial oedema and lymphocyte invasion. Testes: oedema, perivascular lymphocyte invasion, focal haemorrhage, destruction of germinal epithelium and tubular plugging. The CNS, pancreas, ovaries, breasts, thyroid and joints are less frequently involved.
Clinical features	The incubation period of 14–18 days is followed by a generalized febrile illness, sometimes associated with convulsions in small children. Tender parotid or submandibular gland swelling (Figs 13 & 14), bilateral in 70%, surrounded by oedema, lasts for a few days. Meningeal irritation is common. Mumps virus is easily cultured from saliva or CSF. Paired sera show an antibody titre rise.
Complications	• *Orchitis*: incidence 20% of post-pubertal males (Fig. 15). Bilateral orchitis may result in sub-fertility. • *Lymphocytic meningitis*: a frequent cause of viral meningitis during epidemics. • *Post-infectious encephalitis, pancreatitis, oophoritis and thyroiditis*: all rare. • *Arthritis*: infrequent, transient and affecting the larger joints.
Treatment	Symptomatic. NSAIDs may relieve the pain of orchitis.
Prevention	Notifiable in the UK. A safe, live attenuated mumps vaccine (Jeryl Lynn strain) is available for childhood immunization. The Urabe strain vaccine was associated with benign aseptic meningitis in 1 in 5–10 000 recipients and is no longer available. In the UK immunization is accomplished using combined measles/mumps/rubella (MMR) vaccine given between 12–18 months of age.

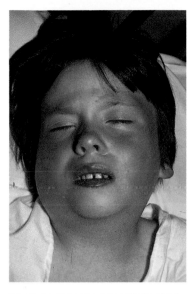

Fig. 13 Parotid and submandibular gland swelling.

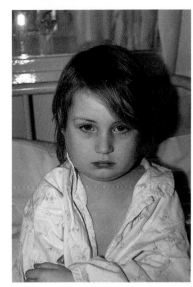

Fig. 14 Mumps parotitis.

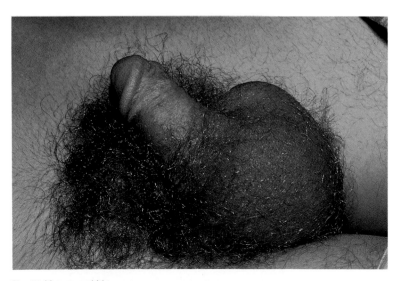

Fig. 15 Mumps orchitis.

Erythema infectiosum (slapped cheek disease)

Aetiology
The human parvovirus B19 (HPV B19).

Incidence
World-wide distribution, most common in children aged 4–15 years.

Pathogenesis
Spread occurs via respiratory droplet emission from active cases. Up to 30% of household contacts are affected. HPV B19 multiplies in rapidly dividing cells, notably red cell precursors (which may lyse). Viraemia follows in 5–7 days. Rash and arthritis result from a host–virus interaction, probably immune-complex mediated. Aplastic crises and haemolytic anaemias may follow erythroid dysplasia. A third of intrauterine HPV B19 infections cause hydrops fetalis or stillbirths.

Clinical features
- *Erythema infectiosum*: the incubation period (5–10 days) is followed by non-tender erythema of the cheeks (Fig. 16) and thereafter by the characteristic lace-like rash over the limbs and trunk (Fig. 17). The rash is more common in older children. These features persist for 7–10 days.
- *Arthritis*: most common in adult contacts, usually producing symmetrical arthralgia lasting several weeks.
- *Aplastic crises*: HPV B19 is the most common cause of aplastic crises in patients with sickle cell anaemia and also causes aplasia in patients with other forms of chronic haemolytic anaemia.
- *Immunodeficient patients*: chronic infection may cause severe persistent anaemia or transient aplasia.

Diagnosis
Serology for specific IgM and IgG antibodies is available but culture for HPV B19 is not normally undertaken.

Treatment and prevention
Treatment is symptomatic: arthritis responds to NSAIDs. Experimental vaccines may be developed for human use. Parvovirus vaccines are in widespread use in animals.

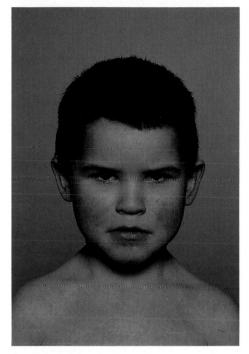

Fig. 16 Erythema infectiosum (slapped cheek appearance).

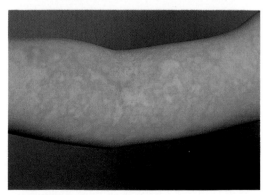

Fig. 17 Typical lace-like skin rash (adult).

Chickenpox

Aetiology

Varicella-zoster virus: a DNA containing herpes virus. *Synonyms*: varicella, herpes zoster.

Incidence

World-wide distribution in those areas where immunization is not routinely applied: more common in children after 9 months, with clusters in winter and early spring. Maternal antibody acquired in utero protects younger infants. Less common but more severe in adults. Congenital and neonatal chickenpox are rare but may be severe.

Pathogenesis

Highly infectious: airborne droplet transmission from active cases of chickenpox and, less commonly, skin scales and exudates in shingles. Histologically identical skin lesions occur in the middle and deep epidermis in both chickenpox and shingles. Cell damage produces oedema which forms clear vesicle fluid. This transforms into a cloudy pustule after WBC invade and then a scab which separates leaving a fine papery scar. Chickenpox rarely causes a haemorrhagic, oedematous, necrotic pneumonia more common and severe in immunocompromised patients. Miliary calcification may follow. Encephalitis is rare.

Keratitis and corneal ulcers are seen less often than with H. simplex infections. Haemorrhagic chickenpox results from thrombocytopenia and DIC.

Clinical features

The incubation period of 2 weeks (range 7–23 days) may be followed by an initial influenza-like illness in adults but the rash (Figs 18 & 19) is often present from the outset, commonly with little fever in children. Commencing as macules, the rash becomes vesicular, then pustular and crusting unless aborted by antiviral agents. Crops of spots occur every day or two (Fig. 20). The scalp, face and trunk are more affected than the limbs and prominences and there is an accompanying enanthem (Fig. 21). The rash is often sparse in children but may be profuse in adults and immunocompromised patients (see Fig. 22, p. 16). Uncomplicated chickenpox lasts about 7 days. Diagnosis is confirmed by virus isolation from vesicle fluid and rising antibody titres.➤

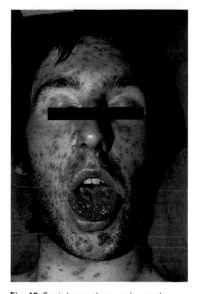

Fig. 18 Facial exanthem and enanthem on tongue.

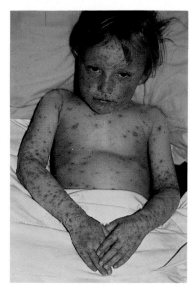

Fig. 19 Distribution in eczematous child (atypical).

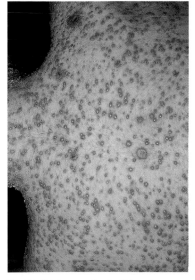

Fig. 20 Chickenpox (varicella) rash: note cropping of lesions.

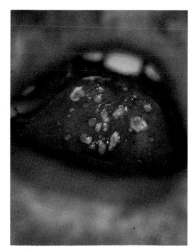

Fig. 21 Palatal enanthem.

Acquired complications	<ul><li>*Common*: Secondary bacterial infection with penetrating septic lesions or</li><li>*Rare*: (a) *varicella pneumonia* (Figs 23 & 24), usually seen in healthy young adults, severe disease occurs in neonates, the elderly or immunodeficient (b) *cerebellitis* and other *encephalopathies*, characterized by ataxia and nystagmus and, more rarely, coma. (c) *varicella gangrenosa* (Fig. 25)</li><li>*Herpes zoster* (shingles): after primary chickenpox, varicella-zoster virus remains dormant in the dorsal spinal horn of peripheral sensory nerves. Reactivations cause zoster which may affect one-third of patients aged >60 years.</li></ul>
Congenital varicella syndrome	Maternal acquisition of varicella in early pregnancy may cause fetal brain and limb defects. Risk of severe involvement is less than 1 in 200 affected pregnancies. Efficacy of hyper-immune globulin in prevention after exposure is unproven. Termination of pregnancy is rarely advised (cf. congenital rubella syndrome).
Treatment	Management is largely symptomatic. Secondary skin sepsis, usually caused by staphylococci or streptococci, may require oral flucloxacillin or macrolide (erythromycin) treatment. Intravenous aciclovir, a nucleoside antiviral agent, is highly effective in severe infections in neonates or the immunosuppressed. It is not used routinely in childhood infections. Aciclovir does not eradicate neurologically-sequestered, non-replicating virus or prevent reactivational zoster (shingles).
Prevention	Patients should be isolated from non-immune or immunocompromised patients. Zoster immune globulin may prevent disease in vulnerable contacts. Live attenuated vaccines are of variable immunogenicity and reactogenicity, but children usually respond well. More widespread use of vaccine is probable.

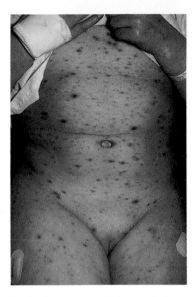

Fig. 22 Haemorrhagic chickenpox in acute leukaemia.

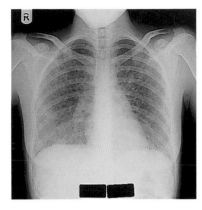

Fig. 23 Chickenpox (varicella) pneumonia.

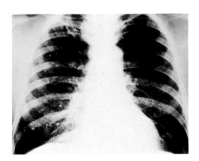

Fig. 24 Chickenpox pneumonia: late calcification.

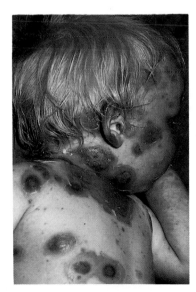

Fig. 25 Varicella gangrenosa.

2 / Herpes zoster (shingles)

Aetiology

The varicella-zoster (V-Z) virus: a DNA containing herpes virus.

Incidence

World-wide distribution (as chickenpox) but no seasonal variation. Common in the elderly (30% incidence in those aged >60 years), rare in childhood.

Pathogenesis

Skin lesions in H. zoster are histologically identical to chickenpox but follow sensory cranial or peripheral nerve root distributions with inflammation and necrosis of ganglion cells. Motor cells are infrequently affected. Widespread lesions occur in the immunocompromised. V-Z virus is neurotropic, often lying dormant in CNS tissue for many years after childhood chickenpox, until reactivated. Reactivation can complicate immunosuppression due to malignancy, corticosteroid and cytotoxic drugs or radiotherapy but such precipitants are usually absent. Shingles is less infectious than chickenpox.

Clinical features

Burning pain or paraesthesiae in the affected dermatome is the usual presenting feature. Pain can be mild or severe and of short or long duration, sometimes being replaced by protracted post-herpetic neuralgia. A day or so after the pain starts, skin lesions appear, confined to the affected dermatome with evolution from macule, through vesicle, pustule, crust and scar as in chickenpox. Vesiculo-pustular lesions often coalesce. A girdle-like eruption following a unilateral thoracic dermatome is the most common manifestation (Figs 26 & 27), but any sensory nerve can be affected, e.g. ophthalmic division of the trigeminal nerve (Figs 28 & 29) or supraclavicular nerves (see Fig. 30, p. 20). Sacral shingles (see Fig. 31, p. 20) may interfere with bladder and bowel function. Limb girdle or peripheral limb involvement may be associated with mixed motor and sensory disturbance.➡

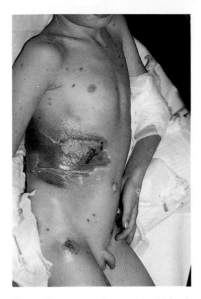

Fig. 26 Herpes zoster (unusual in children).

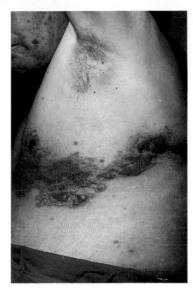

Fig. 27 Fully developed thoracic zoster: limited to single dermatome.

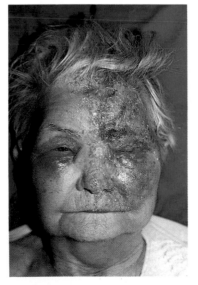

Fig. 28 Early ophthalmic zoster with secondary infection.

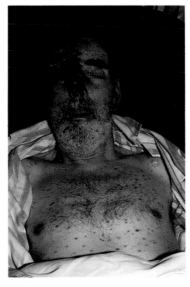

Fig. 29 Late ophthalmic zoster: generalized rash in leukaemia.

Motor and sensory involvement is typical of the Ramsay–Hunt syndrome (Fig. 32) comprising ear pain, vesicles on the external auditory meatus, with facial palsy and loss of taste. Any branch of the trigeminal nerve may be affected, but herpes zoster ophthalmicus is most common. When the nasociliary branch is involved, corneal damage may result. Virus may be grown on tissue culture from the skin lesions. Antibody titres rise during the illness.

A sparse generalized eruption similar to chickenpox may accompany zoster; it may be severe and profuse in immunocompromised patients, notably in lymphoma patients.

Complications

Secondary bacterial infection may occur. In immunocompromised patients extensive disseminated skin lesions resemble chickenpox. Pneumonia and meningoencephalitis are rare. Post-herpetic neuralgia, a common sequel within affected dermatome(s), produces transient but severe attacks of pain, persisting for months.

Treatment

Analgesics are usually required. Secondary staphylococcal or streptococcal infection responds to oral flucloxacillin. Oral aciclovir (800 mg 5 × daily) given early can arrest progression and is useful for ophthalmic, sacral and motor disease. Pharmacologically improved alternatives, such as famciclovir and valaciclovir, allow less frequent dosage and thus encourage compliance. Intravenous aciclovir is often required for severe generalized chickenpox complicating zoster in the elderly and is life saving in immunocompromised patients. Ophthalmic zoster with conjunctival involvement requires IV aciclovir plus topical aciclovir and chloramphenicol to treat secondary bacterial conjunctivitis. Topical homatropine and corticosteroids may be advised by the ophthalmologist. Post-herpetic neuralgia can be refractory but may respond to carbamazepine, transcutaneous nerve stimulation or nerve ablation.

Prevention

Once acquired, V-Z virus may erupt as shingles at any time. This is not preventable. Patients with zoster are infectious and should be isolated.

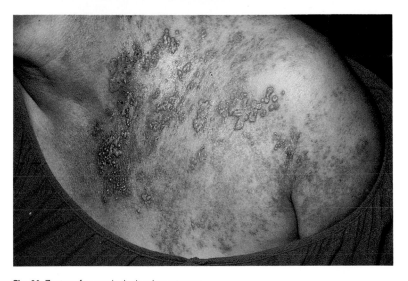

Fig. 30 Zoster of supraclavicular dermatomes.

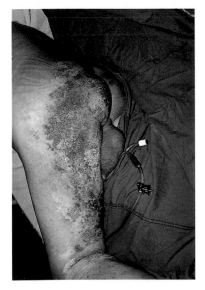

Fig. 31 Sacral shingles.

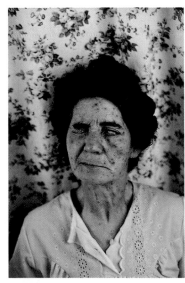

Fig. 32 Ramsay–Hunt syndrome: facial palsy.

3 / Herpes simplex infections

Aetiology

Two DNA-containing viruses, distinguishable epidemiologically, clinically and serologically as Herpes simplex types 1 and 2 (HSV-1 and HSV-2). Synonyms: Herpesvirus hominis I/II.

Incidence

Primary HSV-1 infection is usually acquired in infancy by the airborne droplet route. Congenital infection with HSV-1 is rare. Congenital HSV-2 disease may occur but is less common than perinatal infection acquired from the maternal birth canal. Most HSV-2 infection in adults is sexually acquired especially by male homosexuals and the promiscuous.

Pathogenesis

Non-immune patients are vulnerable to virus shed from the skin and mucosae of active cases over several days. HSV-1 usually affects the mucocutaneous junctions of lips and nose and HSV-2 the genitalia. Virus replication in the epithelium or mucosae causes inflammation, cell lysis and thin walled vesicles. After primary infection, HSV-1 and HSV-2 migrate to nerves where they lie dormant. Reactivation may be precipitated by bacterial infection, e.g. pneumonia (herpes febrilis), sunlight, menstruation and immunosuppression.

Clinical features

Primary HSV-1 stomatitis consists of painful ulcerating vesicles on the lips, anterior buccal mucosa and nares (Figs 33 & 34). Congenital HSV-1 or HSV-2 infection (Fig. 35) causes jaundice, thrombocytopenia, hepatosplenomegaly, rashes, encephalopathy and choroidoretinitis. In eczematous patients HSV-1 infection may be widespread (Kaposi's varicelliform eruption, eczema herpeticum: Fig. 36, p. 24). Similar eruptions may be the presenting features of AIDS (Ch. 38) or of other diseases associated with immunosuppression, e.g. lymphoma.➡

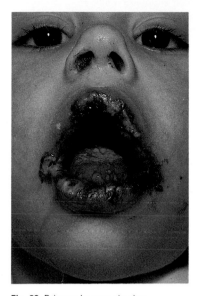

Fig. 33 Primary herpes simplex stomatitis.

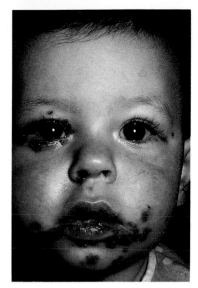

Fig. 34 Primary stomatitis with skin, nasal and periocular involvement.

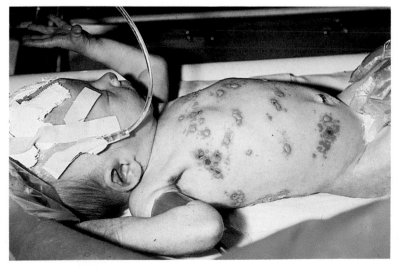

Fig. 35 Congenital disseminated herpes simplex.

Primary HSV-2 infection usually affects the genitalia or anus with clusters of painful vesicles lasting for 10 days (Fig. 37). Health care workers may be infected on the fingers, resulting in herpetic whitlow (Fig. 38). Dendritic corneal ulcers (Fig. 39) can cause blindness and are more common in HSV-1 than HSV-2 infections. HSV-1 encephalitis may complicate neonatal, primary or asymptomatic reactivation of virus with focal CNS signs, confusion and coma. CSF is often normal and culture-negative but CT/MRI brain scans demonstrate focal disease, especially in the temporal lobes.

Virus can be isolated from the infected mouth, anus and genitalia and, in encephalitis, from brain biopsy but usually not from CSF (PCR may become more routinely available). Serology is diagnostic in primary infections but is of little value during reactivations or encephalitis.

Treatment

Most routine HSV-1 skin and mucosal infections are localized and require no specific therapy. Corneal ulceration should be treated with topical aciclovir (steroids are *contraindicated*). Secondary infection by oral anaerobes in stomatitis may benefit from metronidazole.

The period of discomfort and virus shedding from acute HSV-2 lesions is reduced by oral aciclovir. Single courses of aciclovir do not preven subsequent recurrences but extended therapy (for 3 months) can reduce their frequency in patients with regular attacks. Intravenous aciclovir is the treatment of choice in encephalitis and disseminated infection, significantly reducing mortality and residual neurological damage providing it is given early. Famciclovir and valaciclovir are alternatives.

Prevention

Active cases should be isolated from babies and the immunosuppressed. Health care personnel with herpetic whitlows or other active lesions should not work with infants or the immunosuppressed. Sexual activity should be avoided in acute HSV-2 disease. Experimental vaccines are under evaluation.

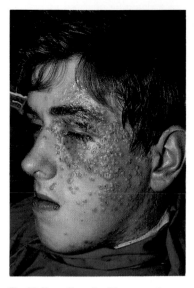

Fig. 36 Kaposi's varicelliform eruption (eczema herpeticum).

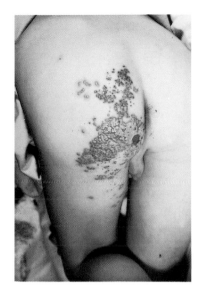

Fig. 37 HSV-2 in a child.

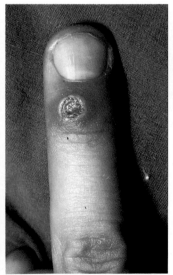

Fig. 38 Herpetic whitlow (surgeon's finger).

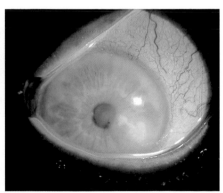

Fig. 39 Dendritic corneal ulcer (H. simplex).

4 / Kawasaki (mucocutaneous lymph node) syndrome

Aetiology	Unknown: presumed transmissable on epidemiological grounds.
Incidence	World-wide, affecting children, particularly Asiatics and blacks. Mini-epidemics occur in winter and spring based on background endemic disease.
Pathogenesis	An immunological reaction to an infectious agent. Immune complexes and activated B cells (producing IgG/IgM) circulate, causing inflammatory vasculitis, resembling infant polyarteritis and affecting joints and coronary arteries.
Clinical features	• *Acute febrile phase*: lasting 7–10 days, characterized by fever of at least 5 days' duration, conjunctivitis, fissuring of lips, mucosal injection, strawberry tongue, swelling of extremities, cervical lymphadenopathy, erythema and rashes (Figs 40 & 41).
	• *Subacute phase*: lasting 2 weeks thereafter with resolution of acute signs. Peripheral desquamation (Fig. 42), accompanied by arthritis and thrombocytosis.
	• *Convalescent phase*: ESR remains elevated for up to 10 weeks. Coronary artery involvement occurs in >20%.
	• *Coronary artery disease*: the prognosis usually good but some develop aneurysm (Fig. 43), stenosis and occlusion (2% mortality). Risk factors include male Caucasians, age <1 year, prolonged fever, high IgE and platelet count, dysrhythmias and cardiomegaly.
Diagnosis	Diagnostic serology is not available. Laboratory findings include leucocytosis, anaemia, high ESR and IgE, and thrombocytosis peaking at 3 weeks. Coronary arteries should be assessed by biplanar echocardiography in phases 2/3.
Treatment and prevention	High-dose aspirin commenced on diagnosis, and reduced in convalescence. Early IV immunoglobulin therapy may prevent coronary artery damage. Corticosteroids are contraindicated.

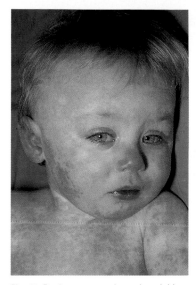

Fig. 40 Erythematous rash, conjunctivitis and sore lips.

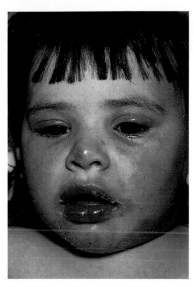

Fig. 41 Kawasaki syndrome: facial rash, cherry red lips, angular stomatitis and conjunctivitis.

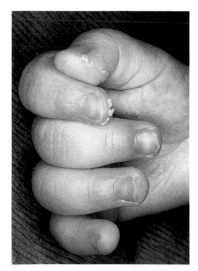

Fig. 42 Peri-ungual desquamation.

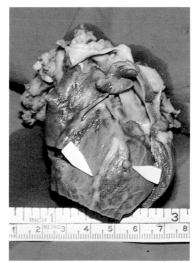

Fig. 43 Kawasaki syndrome: coronary artery aneurysm/stenosis.

5 / Lyme disease

Aetiology	Borrelia burgdorferi, a tick-borne spirochaete.
Incidence	World-wide, related to the distribution of the vector ixodid tick. Seasonal fluctuations in spring/autumn. Seroprevalence of evidence of past infection in rural population may be 5% or more.
Pathogenesis	Haematogenous spread from initial bite infects skin, joints and CNS. Persistent infection plus host-response produces chronic symptoms.
Clinical features	• *Erythema chronicum migrans* (ECM): an expanding, non-painful red maculo-papular eruption (Figs 44 & 45) around the tick-bite. It can reach 10–20 cm in diameter and fades at the centre. Secondary lesions follow at distant sites in 40%. These lesions fade in 3–4 weeks. • *Early disseminated disease*: ECM is accompanied by fever, myalgia, arthralgia and headache in 50%. • *Later manifestations*: 　1. *Oligoarthritis*: >50% will develop transient, recurrent acute arthritis. 　2. *Carditis*: follows in 10%. 　3. *Neuroborreliosis*: neurological involvement follows in 25%. Bell's palsy is an early sign. Meningoencephalitis with cognitive dysfunction, cranial and peripheral neuropathy may all occur.
Diagnosis	Indirect immunofluorescence tests for IgM antibody will be positive after 5–6 weeks. IgG persists long term. PCR may prove more effective. In CNS disease, CSF examination shows a lymphocytic pleocytosis and MRI may confirm encephalitis. Antibody can be detected in CSF.
Treatment and prevention	ECM responds to either doxycycline for 2 weeks or parenteral benzyl penicillin. Ceftriaxone is more effective for CNS involvement. Avoidance of tick-bite is the only form of prevention.

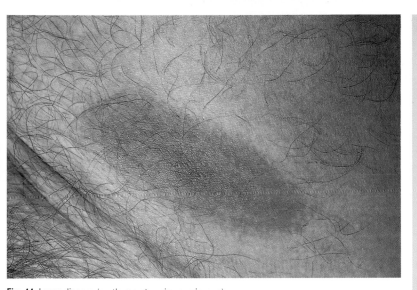

Fig. 44 Lyme disease (erythema chronicum migrans).

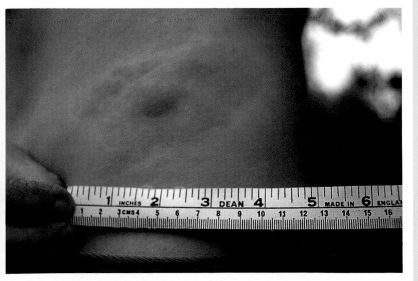

Fig. 45 Lyme disease (erythema chronicum migrans).

Aetiology	Orf virus: an ovoid paravaccinia virus.
Incidence	A common world-wide zoonosis of sheep and goats, causing watery papillomatous lesions on the mucosae and conjunctivae. Man is infected during direct occupational contact with the animal, most commonly during spring lambing. Now rare in UK and many countries due to preventative veterinary vaccines.
Pathogenesis	A nodule appears at the site of the contact where virus enters through a laceration or abrasion of the skin. A vesiculo-bulbous hyperplastic mass develops, usually without further spread.
Clinical features	Shepherds are infected at lambing time but shearers, abbatoir workers and veterinary surgeons can also catch orf. Exposed surfaces such as hands, forearms or the face are usually affected. An irritating but pain-free nodule with a gelatinous appearance (Fig. 46) develops and enlarges. It is often incised (wrongly) but no material can be expressed. Healing (Fig. 47) usually occurs without scarring and takes some weeks. Secondary bacterial cellulitis or lymphangitis may occur. Erythema multiforme is an occasional complication. Virus can be isolated from the lesion and demonstrated by electron microscopy.
Treatment	No specific treatment is available. Oral flucloxacillin or erythromycin are effective for secondary bacterial infection. The lesion should not be incised.
Prevention	Gloves should be worn when handling infected animals. Isolation of patients is unnecessary. An effective ovine vaccine is now available which prevents enzootic disease in sheep.

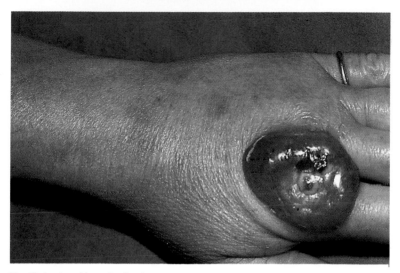

Fig. 46 Acute orf in a shepherdess.

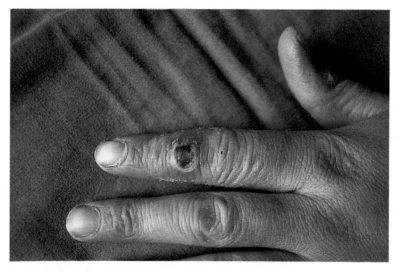

Fig. 47 Healing orf.

7 / Herpangina

Aetiology	Coxsackie A viruses of various types, e.g. 2, 4, 5, 6, 8, 10, 23, less commonly Coxsackie B viruses and Echoviruses.
Incidence	Sporadic, subject to minor epidemic fluctuations. May be accompanied by an upsurge of viral meningitis, enteritis and infantile febrile episodes due to the same epidemic type. Many infections are asymptomatic or trivial.
Pathogenesis	Spreads by the faecal–oral route and, less commonly, via airborne droplet emission, usually in primary schoolchildren who transmit infection to older siblings and parents.
Clinical features	Herpangina is characterized by acute onset, fever, moderate systemic toxaemia and ulcerative pharyngitis (Fig. 48). Fluctuant pyrexia is present initially accompanied by ulcers of the palatal pillars, posterior soft palate and uvula, and, less commonly, of the tonsils and posterior aspect of the tongue. Complicating parotitis has been described. Ulcers are 1–5 mm in size, covered by necrotic slough and spare the anterior of the mouth—in contrast with herpes simplex stomatitis and Stevens–Johnson syndrome. There is no accompanying rash. Resolution may take up to a week. Diagnosis is primarily clinical, supported by virus isolation from throat and stool. Serology may reveal a diagnostic rise in antibody titre.
Treatment	Non specific, antibiotics are not indicated. Symptomatic relief may be obtained with aspirin gargles.
Prevention	Isolation not usually necessary. No specific preventative measures are available.

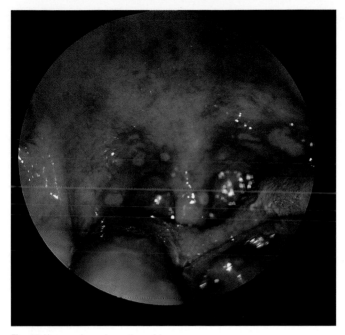

Fig. 48 Herpangina: ulceration of fauces.

8 / Hand, foot and mouth disease

Aetiology	Coxsackie virus A16 (occasionally A5 or A10).
Incidence	This unusual manifestation of enteroviral activity is associated with clusters of clinical cases when infection is widespread in the community. Virus is often isolated from asymptomatic family contacts. World-wide distribution but probably more common in temperate zones.
Pathogenesis	Spreads primarily by faecal–oral transmission from active cases and convalescent excretors: probably also by the airborne droplet route from active cases. Viraemia is followed by a typically distributed peripheral skin rash and accompanying oral lesions.
Clinical features	The incubation period of 3–7 days is followed by the appearance of bright red spots or small vesicles on the buccal mucosa, which ulcerate and then heal within 7–10 days. These ulcers are painful and affect mainly the lips, tongue, buccal mucosa and palate but spare the back of the throat. A sparse, painless rash of the hands and feet affects the lateral aspects of fingers and toes but also involves the palms and soles. In infancy the buttocks may be affected. Skin lesions (Figs 49 & 50) vary from red macules to small vesicles containing milky fluid and bullae which ulcerate and heal 7–10 days later. In children, mild fever and malaise are common: adults have little systemic upset. There are no specific complications. Virus can be isolated by tissue culture or material from oral and skin lesions. Specific serum antibodies show a diagnostic rise in titre.
Treatment	Management is symptomatic only. Antibiotics are not indicated.
Prevention	Good hygiene, although by the time of diagnosis other household members will already be infected, whether symptomatic or not.

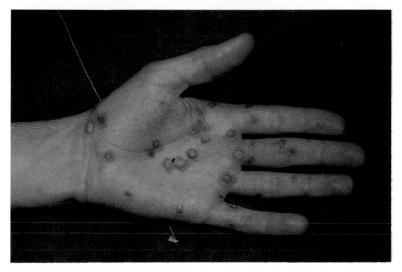

Fig. 49 Palmar vesicles.

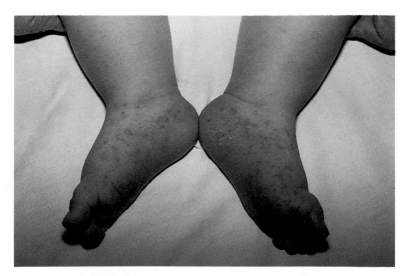

Fig. 50 Milky vesicles on feet.

9/ Infectious mononucleosis (IM)

Aetiology	Epstein–Barr virus (EBV), a herpes virus. Similar illness caused by toxoplasmosis, cytomegalovirus infection and primary HIV infection.
Incidence	World-wide distribution causing glandular fever (Europe and N. America). EBV is also associated with Burkitt's lymphoma (Africa) and nasopharyngeal carcinoma (Far East). Subclinical infection with seroconversion is common. Glandular fever is most common in adolescents.
Pathogenesis	Close contact and kissing facilitate transmission of EBV from saliva of both cases and, more often, asymptomatic individuals. After oropharyngeal invasion, virus infects B-lymphocytes which form heterophile antibody. Some B-cells are transformed and EBV-containing B-cells continue to replicate. Next, killer T-cells destroy some EBV infected B-cells and suppressor T-cells limit B-cell transformation. The T-cell response causes the lymph node and splenic enlargement, anginose (painful, choking) sore throat and the characteristic atypical lymphocytes seen in the peripheral blood. Later a long lasting balance ensues between infected B-cells and killer T-cells. If transformed B-cells proliferate, in the absence of T-cells, or if virus overwhelms B-cells causing agammaglobulinaemia, fulminating disease results.
Clinical features	The incubation period of 4–8 weeks is followed by an illness of 2–3 weeks' duration, characterized by sore throat, malaise, a swinging and hectic fever, splenomegaly and generalized tender lymphadenopathy. Pus and pseudomembrane cover the tonsils (Fig. 51) but clear in 1–2 weeks. Periorbital oedema (Fig. 52) and cervical lymphadenopathy (see Fig. 54, p. 38) are prominent and palatal petechiae are typical (Fig. 53). Hepatomegaly and mild jaundice, and a pink maculopapular rash occur less commonly (see Figs 55 & 56, p. 38). Life-long immunity is conferred.➡

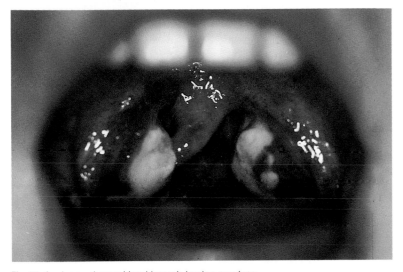

Fig. 51 Anginose pharyngitis with wash-leather exudate.

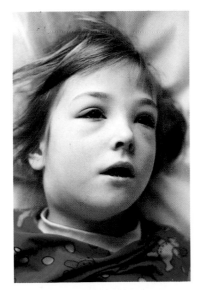

Fig. 52 Facial oedema and cervical lymphadenopathy.

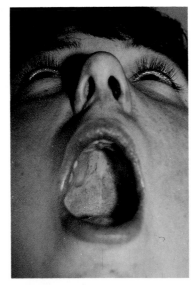

Fig. 53 Palatal petechiae.

Diagnosis	Atypical mononuclear cells are present in the peripheral blood and the Monospot slide test and Paul Bunnell test for IgG antibodies are positive. Rising titres of EBV specific IgG antibody and IgM antibody, which reflects acute infection, can be demonstrated. Liver function tests indicate mild hepatocellular damage.
Complications	*Splenic rupture, airway obstruction, blood dyscrasias* or *CNS complications* may occasionally prove fatal. *Haemolysis, thrombocytopenia, pneumonitis, encephalitis, meningitis, post-infectious polyneuropathy, lymphoma* and *myocarditis* may occur. Administration of ampicillin or amoxycillin characteristically causes a maculopapular skin rash 7–8 days after start of therapy (Fig. 56). *Transient depression* is a common sequel. Glandular fever is one of the frequent antecedent causes of *post-viral fatigue* and the *chronic fatigue syndrome (myalgic encephalomyelitis)*.
Treatment	Adequate rest is important. Ganciclovir therapy may globally improve symptoms but its value remains unproven in routine cases. Prednisolone or emergency tracheostomy are sometimes required for severe pharyngeal oedema causing incipient respiratory obstruction. Superimposed streptococcal infection is treated with penicillin or erythromycin. Ampicillin or amoxycillin are contraindicated. Complicating haemolytic anaemia usually responds to prednisolone and transfusion.
Prevention	No active or passive immunization is available. Strict isolation is not necessary.

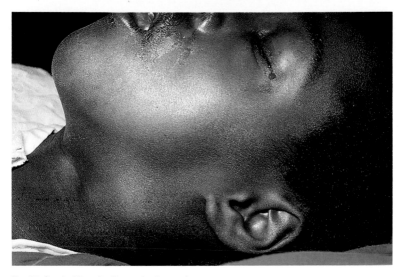

Fig. 54 Cervical lymphadenopathy (severe).

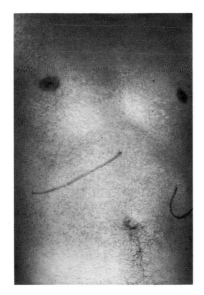

Fig. 55 Rash and hepatosplenomegaly.

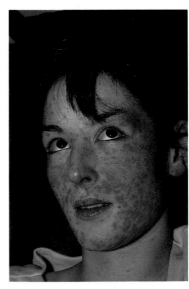

Fig. 56 Jaundice and ampicillin rash.

10 / Toxoplasmosis

Aetiology	*Toxoplasma gondii*, an intracellular protozoon parasite.
Incidence	Asymptomatic infection common in immuno-competent subjects: severe CNS disease may follow re-activation in AIDS. Congenital infection occurs in 0.1% of live births.
Pathogenesis	A zoonosis, primarily a disease of cats but also of intermediates such as birds. Acquired by ingestion of oocysts, commonly from kitten faeces, or by airborne droplet transmission. Disseminates in reticuloendothelial and other tissues. Latent infection and transplacental fetal spread may follow.

Clinical features	• *Acquired disease*. A mononucleosis syndrome characterized by fever, atypical mononucleosis lymphadenopathy and splenomegaly is common. Choroidoretinitis and encephalitis are rare.
	 • *Congenital disease*
	   1. *Disseminated syndrome*: features include jaundice, lymphadenopathy, splenomegaly and choroidoretinitis (Figs 57 & 58).
	   2. *Neurological*: hydrocephalus, convulsions, intracranial calcification (Fig. 59). Perinatal mortality is 10–20%.
	 • *Opportunistic disease*. Reactivation of latent infection in immunosuppressed patients may cause severe encephalitis, e.g. in AIDS patients.

Diagnosis	Toxoplasmosis is diagnosed serologically by the Sabin–Feldman dye test and IgM titres. In encephalitis, CT scan shows focal ring-enhanced lesions (see Fig. 169, p. 122).
Treatment	Severe disease is treated with high dose sulfadiazine and pyrimethamine plus folinic acid. Clindamycin may prove useful and prophylactic spiramycin may reduce materno-fetal transmission. Steroid therapy is of value in choroidoretinitis.
Prevention	Not notifiable: isolation not necessary. No adequate control measures are available but pregnant women should avoid exposure to kittens.

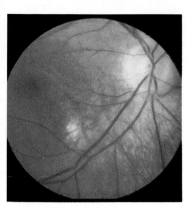

Fig. 57 Acute choroidoretinitis.

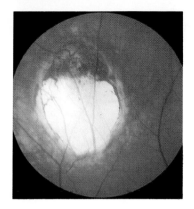

Fig. 58 Healed choroidoretinitis.

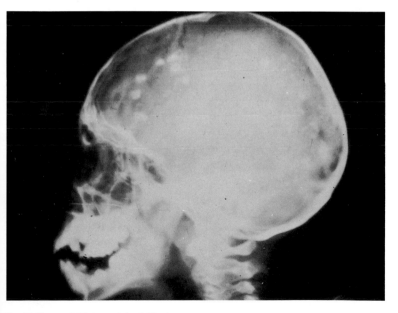

Fig. 59 Congenital intracranial calcification.

11 / Cytomegalovirus infection

Aetiology	Cytomegalovirus: a DNA containing herpes virus.
Incidence	World-wide distribution. Most infections are subclinical but many symptomatic intrauterine, neonatal and adult acquired infections occur. Peaks of incidence occur between 1 and 2 years and 15–30 years.
Pathogenesis	Spreads by airborne droplet transmission from infected nasopharyngeal secretions. Transplacental infection may arise from primary infection or reactivation of latent virus during pregnancy. Perinatal infection results from maternal cervical infection. Infected infants excrete virus in the urine for months. CMV infected cells swell and show intranuclear and intracytoplasmic inclusions. Nuclear chromatin is pushed to the edge of the cell giving an "owl's eye" appearance (Fig. 60).
Clinical features	• *Congenital CMV disease* (Fig. 62): choroidoretinitis, hepatosplenomegaly, jaundice, rash, microcephaly and deafness.
	• *Acquired CMV disease*: is clinically indistinguishable from infectious mononucleosis although membranous pharyngitis is uncommon. Choroidoretinitis may occur. In immunosuppressed (tumour/transplant) patients primary or reactivational CMV pneumonitis has a mortality of >50%.
	• *AIDS*: CMV retinitis (Fig. 61), pneumonitis and colitis are common. Diagnosis is established by virus isolation from tissues, urine and saliva and a rising antibody titre. An atypical lymphocytosis is usually found in peripheral blood.
Treatment	IV ganciclovir or foscarnet may control but neither eliminates CMV disease in AIDS or immunocompromised patients.
Prevention	Vaccine in development. Transfusion of CMV antibody-negative blood is recommended for immunocompromised and HIV-infected patients.

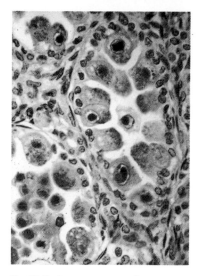

Fig. 60 Owl's eye appearance in toxoplasmosis.

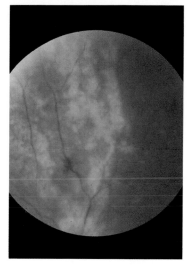

Fig. 61 CMV retinitis in AIDS patient.

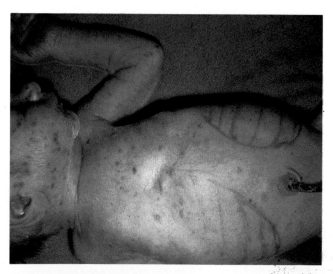

Fig. 62 Congenital rash and hepatomegaly.

Aetiology	Viruses of hepatitis A, B, C (HAV, HBV, HCV), delta agent, hepatitis E (HEV), hepatitis G (HGV, a flavivirus, formerly non A-E virus). EBV (Ch. 9), cytomegalovirus (Ch. 11), HSV I/II (Ch. 3) and haemorrhagic fever viruses are also hepatotropic.
Incidence	World-wide distribution. HAV affects the young and is often subclinical. HBV, uncommon in the West, except in homosexuals and addicts, is prevalent in Africa and the Far East. HEV is uncommon outside the Indian subcontinent.
Pathogenesis	HAV and HEV are transmitted by the faecal-oral route. Neither causes chronic disease but HEV is dangerous in pregnancy. HCV and HGV are spread by infusion of unscreened blood products, HBV by sexual and parenteral routes from cases and carriers. Delta agent usually requires the presence of hepatitis B surface antigen (HBsAg) for pathogenicity. Simultaneous delta and HBV infection cause *brisk* hepatitis. Delta infection in HBV carriers may precipitate fulminant or chronic aggressive hepatitis. HBV, HCV and HGV can be transmitted vertically: all three may cause chronic hepatitis. HBV is associated with hepatocellular carcinoma. Viral hepatitis causes centrilobular necrosis and portal inflammation.
Clinical features	Approximate incubation periods are: HAV 15–40 days, HBV 50–140 days, HCV and HGV 30–160 days, delta and HEV 30–90 days. Illness starts with malaise, nausea, vomiting, mild fever and abdominal discomfort. Arthralgia may herald hepatitis B. A week later, after the onset of dark urine and pale stools, jaundice appears (Fig. 63). In hepatitis B, evidence of IV drug misuse may be present (Fig. 64). Altered consciousness, a flapping tremor and fetor hepaticus precede complicating coma (Fig. 65). Acute hepatic failure due to fulminant hepatitis has a mortality of 90% due to haemorrhage, cerebral oedema and overwhelming infection.

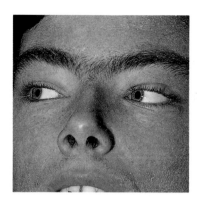

Fig. 63 Jaundice of skin and sclerae.

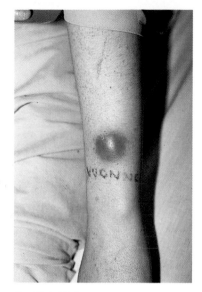

Fig. 64 Addict's arm: tattoo, needle track and abscess.

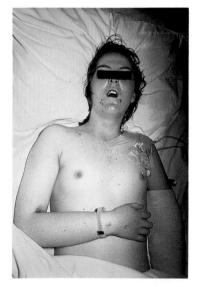

Fig. 65 Terminal hepatic coma: note bruising.

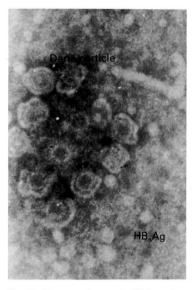

Fig. 66 Electron micrograph: HB$_s$Ag and Dane particles (whole virus) in serum.

Diagnosis	Acute infection is confirmed by HAV-specific IgM response, by demonstration of HBsAg (see Fig. 66, p. 44) and anti-HBc antibody in HBV infection, and by detection of anti-HCV, anti-delta and anti-HEV antibodies as appropriate. PCR-based tests being developed, notably for HGV infection. Typical serological responses in HAV, HBV and HCV infections are summarized in Graphs 1, 2 and 3. Persistence of HBe antigen suggests development of chronic HBV disease.
Treatment	Largely symptomatic in acute disease. Incipient hepatic coma is treated in specialist units with a liver failure regime directed at the complications of cerebral oedema, haemorrhage and fulminant infection. Assessment for liver transplantation may be appropriate. Alpha-interferon is useful in chronic HCV infection.
Prevention	Notification, isolation, screening of blood products and education of high-risk groups. Active HAV immunization is available. Immunoglobulin is used for prophylaxis after known exposure to HAV or HBV. Active HBV immunization is recommended for health care workers and, with anti-HBV immunoglobulin, for neonates of HBsAg positive mothers.

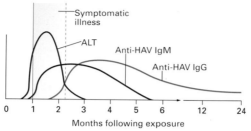

Graph 1. Typical responses in acute HAV hepatitis.

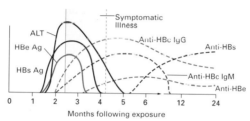

Graph 2. Typical responses in acute self-limiting HBV hepatitis.

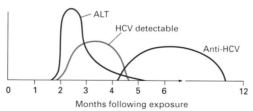

Graph 3. Typical responses in acute self limiting HCV hepatitis.

Aetiology	*Leptospira icterohaemorrhagiae, L. hebdomadis* and *L. canicola*: pathogenic spirochaetes.
Incidence	About 100 cases/year in the UK, similar order of frequency in Europe, more common in Tropics. Occupational risks related to rat-infested environments.
Pathogenesis	Zoonosis from rats (*L. icterohaemorrhagiae*), cattle (*L. hebdomadis*) and dogs or pigs (*L. canicola*), usually by skin contact with urine of infected animals. Produces multisystem disease including hepatitis, nephritis, meningitis, coagulopathies and immune-complex disease.
Clinical features	• *Weil's disease* (*L. icterohaemorrhagiae*): prodromal headache, myalgia, pyrexia, rigors and prostration are followed 1 week later by hepatitis, nephritis, and haemorrhage caused by DIC. Haemorrhagic herpes labialis and subconjunctival haemorrhages are often present (Fig. 67). Agglutination tests, urine cultures and dark ground examination (Fig. 68) are usually diagnostic. • *L. hebdomadis infection*: a milder form of Weil's disease, often with lymphocytic meningitis. • *Canicola fever* (*L. canicola*): prodromal syndrome similar to but less severe than Weil's disease, followed by lymphocytic meningitis.
Complications	Hepatorenal failure causes death in 10% of patients with Weil's disease. Transverse myelitis, uveitis and myopericarditis may occur.
Treatment	Benzyl penicillin or tetracycline are most effective when given in the prodromal phase but may still be effective in symptomatic disease.
Prevention	Notification required in some countries: isolation not necessary. Veterinary vaccines (e.g. Canicola fever) and hygiene in farms, abbatoirs and kennels are important. Tetracycline prophylaxis prevents infection in those exposed to blood or urine.

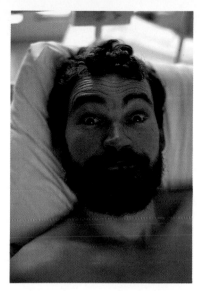

Fig. 67 Facial appearance: jaundice, subconjunctival haemorrhage, haemorrhagic herpes labialis in Weil's disease.

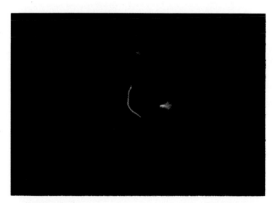

Fig. 68 Leptospirae (dark ground examination of urine).

Aetiology

Coagulase-positive *Staphylococcus aureus*. The skin commensal *Staph. epidermidis* may infect prostheses and ventriculo-atrial shunts, and is also associated with urinary tract infection in sexually active young women.

Incidence

World-wide. Opportunistic infections occur in immunocompromised patients and diabetics.

Pathogenesis

Pathogenic staphylococci are carried on skin or anterior nares and may cause endogenous or exogenous infection by invasion, toxin production or both. Staphylococci enter skin breaches or hair follicles causing local sepsis, polymorphonuclear leucocytosis and pus formation. Invasion of bronchial mucosa devitalised by influenza leads to staphylococcal pneumonia. Superficial skin infections may result in bacteraemia with endocarditis and widespread sepsis. Toxin production or absorption of pre-formed toxin can cause enterotoxin food poisoning (often from milk, dairy products and meat), tampon-associated toxin shock syndrome and exfoliatin induced toxic epidermal necrolysis (TEN), most patients having no detectable TSST-1 antibody.

Clinical features

- *Skin infections*: impetigo (Fig. 69) affects only the superficial epidermis: it is highly infectious. A boil (Fig. 70) is simply an inflamed infected hair follicle from which pus may discharge spontaneously. Coalescence of infected follicles results in a carbuncle. In cellulitis (Fig. 71), the subcutaneous tissues are also infected.
- *Bacteraemia*: results from superficial or deep sepsis or from direct injection of staphylococci by drug addicts. *Endocarditis* may follow with widespread septic emboli to brain, lungs, skin (Fig. 72) and kidneys. Valvular disruption may produce intractable cardiac failure. Pneumonia commonly results in empyema and lung abscesses, notably in cystic fibrosis. Blood cultures are mandatory for diagnosis.➡

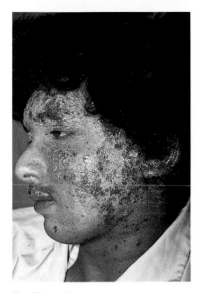

Fig. 69 Impetigo.

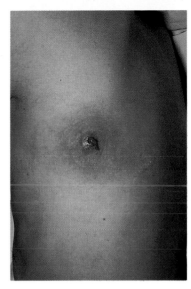

Fig. 70 Boil exuding yellow pus.

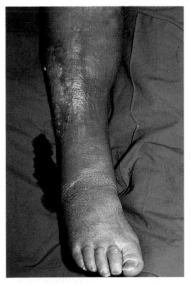

Fig. 71 Cellulitis with epidermal necrosis.

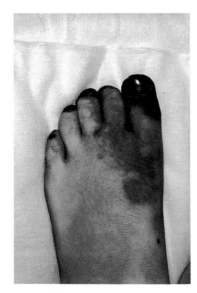

Fig. 72 Septic embolic gangrene in endocarditis.

- *Toxin-induced disease*:
  1. *Food poisoning*: causes profuse vomiting, hypovolaemia, hypotension and prostration, usually without diarrhoea commencing 1–2 h after ingestion of pre-formed staphylococcal enterotoxin.
  2. *Exotoxin-A induced toxic or tampon shock*: is characterized by fever, hypotension and rash. Staphylococci are isolated from the vagina but rarely from blood.
  3. *Toxic epidermal necrolysis* (*TEN*): infants with scalded skin syndrome (Ritter's disease: Figs 73 & 74) or children with Lyell's syndrome (Fig. 75) develop painful erythematous shearing of superficial epidermal bullae. TEN also occurs in immunocompromised adults (Fig. 76).

Diagnosis

Blood cultures are mandatory to detect invasive disease. Anti-staphylolysin titres are unreliable.

Treatment

Superficial skin sepsis is treated with dressings, poultices or surgical drainage. Deeper or systemic infection requires urgent parenteral chemotherapy usually with flucloxacillin plus either fusidic acid or clindamycin. Staphylococcal endocarditis is treated with high dose flucloxacillin plus either fusidic acid (for 4 weeks) or gentamicin (for first week only). Valve replacement is frequently required. Surgical drainage of septic arthritis, lung abscess and empyema may also be necessary. Methicillin-resistant *Staph. aureus* (MRSA) causes hospital outbreaks requiring treatment with vancomycin (resistance reported in Japan).

Prevention

Scrupulous hand washing; asepsis in surgery and with neonates; cleansing of wounds; isolation and/or treatment of MRSA carriers/patients; improved food hygiene. Patients transferred from hospitals with epidemic MRSA should be isolated. Mupirocin may reduce nasal carriage of MRSA.

Control of outbreaks (MRSA)

An infection control team should identify the epidemic strain (phage typing, etc.), trace affected patients/areas, isolate colonized or infected patients, enforce barrier precautions, screen contacts, treat carrier sites, restrict patient and staff movements to other areas and arrange disinfection policies.

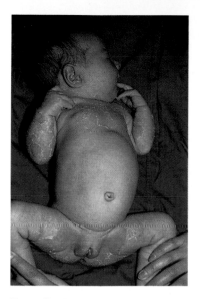

Fig. 73 Ritter's disease.

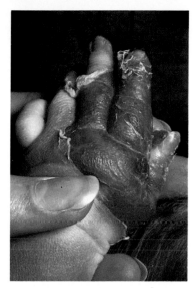

Fig. 74 Ritter's disease.

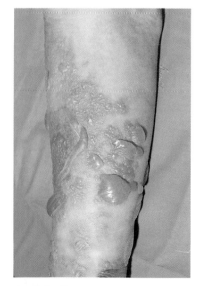

Fig. 75 Lyell's syndrome.

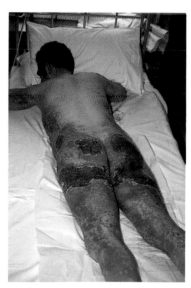

Fig. 76 Toxic epidermal necrolysis (lymphoma patient).

15 / Osteomyelitis (OM)

Aetiology

Staphylococcus aureus causes 80% of cases of OM, most of the remainder being due to *Strep. pyogenes, H. influenzae* and, less commonly, Salmonella, Pseudomonas spp. and TB.

Incidence

Primary staphylococcal OM is most common in males aged 3–10 years. World-wide but more common in those with sickle cell disease and diabetes mellitus and prosthetic joints.

Pathogenesis

During bacteraemia, often asymptomatic, staphylococci settle in metaphyses or sites of bone injury. >60% of staphylococcal OM occurs in the lower limbs. Local inflammation leads to pus formation, periosteal elevation and bone necrosis. 1–2% of hip and knee prostheses suffer complicating infection with loosening, pain and chronic sinus formation. Amyloidosis may complicate chronic disease.

Clinical features

A history of injury may be given. The onset is sudden; with fever, rigors and exquisitely tender local inflammation in the bone or joint. Untreated, septic sinus formation (Fig. 77), bone necrosis leading to sequestrum formation and pathological fracture occur. Pathogens are identified in blood (50–60% positive), bone biopsy and joint fluid cultures. Leucocytosis is usual. Antistaphylolysin titres may assist in chronic disease. X-ray changes, initially calcification under periosteal elevation (Fig. 78) followed by cortical erosion, takes two weeks to develop. Extensive bone destruction may follow (Fig. 79). Isotope bone scanning (Fig. 80) is often diagnostic.

Treatment

Antibiotics are given for 6 weeks. Clindamycin, fusidic acid and flucloxacillin give good results in staphylococcal OM. Chronic disease may require 1–2 years' treatment. Oral ciprofloxacin or IV cephalosporins, e.g. ceftazidime, are useful for Gram-negative and pseudomonal OM. Surgical procedures are required in 50%.

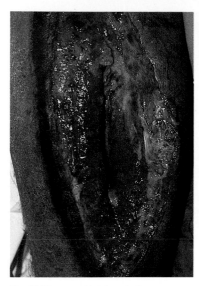

Fig. 77 Sinus on thigh (surgical osteomyelitis).

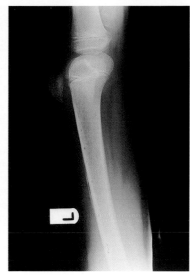

Fig. 78 Early acute osteomyelitis: calcified raised periosteum (lucent zones in anterior tibia from surgical exploration).

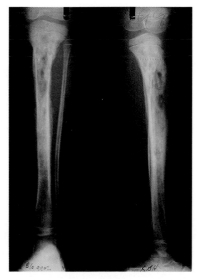

Fig. 79 Late osteomyelitis: extensive bone destruction and sequestrum formation.

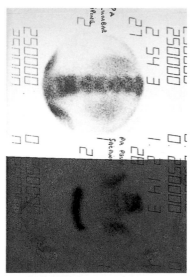

Fig. 80 Multifocal spinal osteomyelitis: isotope bone scan.

Aetiology	Beta-haemolytic streptococci: classified by cell wall carbohydrates into Lancefield's groups and by T-proteins into Griffith's types.
Incidence	World-wide distribution. Pyoderma mainly affects children with poor hygiene in the tropics. Scarlet fever, rheumatic fever and post-streptococcal glomerulonephritis had, until recently, become rare except in the developing world. However, a resurgence of rheumatic fever is currently being encountered in some areas of the industrialized world, including the southern USA.
Pathogenesis	Streptococcal infections, dependent on type, may be highly infectious. Both asymptomatic carriers and those with active disease spread group A infection by airborne droplet transmission. Acquisition is followed by pharyngitis, follicular tonsillitis and cervical adenitis. Skin infection is facilitated by hyaluronidase which assists pyoderma to spread and involve deeper tissues, producing erysipelas and cellulitis. Lymphatic spread may precede bacteraemia. Erythema nodosum, and later rheumatic fever and glomerulonephritis, are immunological reactions to streptococcal infection. Neonates acquire group B haemolytic streptococci from the birth canal and may develop septicaemia (within 5 days) or later septicaemia and meningitis.
Clinical features	• *Erysipelas*: streptococcal invasion of the skin may result in a butterfly facial rash (Figs 81 & 82), or a spreading eruption on a limb, usually the legs, characterized by a red, swollen, painful epidermal lesion with a well demarcated raised edge. Bullae may form.
	• *Pyoderma*: type 49 streptococci cause epidemics of skin sepsis with yellow crusts (Fig. 83), which may be followed by acute glomerulonephritis.
	• *Ascending lymphangitis*: represents tender red inflamed lymph channels (Fig. 84) draining a sometimes unapparent streptococcal infection. Associated bacteraemia may prove fatal.

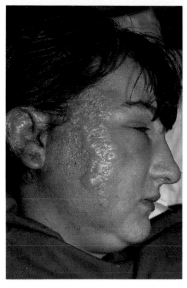

Fig. 81 Facial erysipelas with superficial bullae.

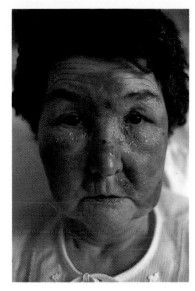

Fig. 82 Healing erysipelas: note raised edge.

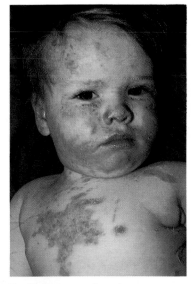

Fig. 83 Streptococcal pyoderma.

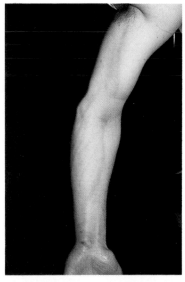

Fig. 84 Ascending lymphangitis from wound at wrist.

- *Pharyngitis, tonsillitis and quinsy*: after 2–4 days' incubation, sore throat, fever, tachycardia and malaise are associated with pharyngitis or follicular tonsillitis (Fig. 85) and cervical adenitis. A bulging peritonsillar abscess or "quinsy" (Fig. 86) may follow. More rarely, suppurative adenitis, sinusitis, otitis media or mastoiditis develop. Viral pharyngitis, glandular fever and diphtheria must be differentiated.
- *Ludwig's angina*: a synergistic infection of the submandibular space (see Figs 87 & 88, p. 60), involving oral microaerophilic streptococci and frequently *Strep. pyogenes*. It may follow dental extraction in immunocompromised patients and can cause airways obstruction.
- *Henoch–Schönlein purpura*: affecting the buttocks and legs (see Fig. 89, p. 60), and associated with arthritis and intestinal colic or bleeding. In childhood, streptococcal infection is the common precipitant. Purpura is vascular in type: thrombocytopenia is absent.
- *Erythema nodosum*: may complicate acute streptococcal infection, tuberculosis, sarcoidosis and drug therapy. Tender, red, raised lumps develop on the shins or elbows (Ch. 33).
- *Rheumatic fever*: onset 2–3 weeks post streptococcal infection and characterized by systemic upset, pyrexia, skin involvement, arthritis and cardiac complications. Diagnosis is confirmed by evidence of recent streptococcal disease plus two major criteria or one major plus two minor criteria, including:
    1. *Major criteria*: carditis, polyarthritis, chorea, erythema marginatum (see Fig. 90, p. 60) and subcutaneous nodules.
    2. *Minor criteria*: fever, joint pain, high ESR or C-reactive protein, leucocytosis, prolonged P-R interval and a past history of rheumatic fever.
  Late cardiovascular sequelae of rheumatic fever include mitral and aortic valve disease with atrial fibrillation and cardiac failure, and bacterial endocarditis.

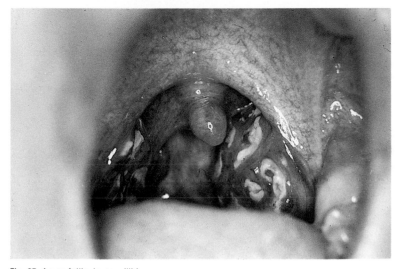

Fig. 85 Acute follicular tonsillitis.

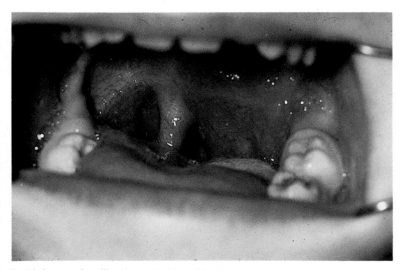

Fig. 86 Acute peritonsillar abscess (quinsy) with trismus.

- *Glomerulonephritis*: group A, type 12 or type 49 (during an epidemic of pyoderma) beta-haemolytic streptococcal infections may be followed by fever, oedema, hypertension and oliguria, proteinuria, haematuria and casts in the urine.

Diagnosis

Beta-haemolytic streptococci may be isolated from the throat, saliva or skin. Blood cultures are commonly positive in acute septic syndromes, e.g. erysipelas and lymphangitis. Serology reveals a rising titre of anti-streptolysin O. A polymorphonuclear leucocytosis and high ESR are usual.

Treatment

Benzyl penicillin is advised initially for most infections but may be followed by oral penicillin-V or amoxycillin in convalescence. Skin infections which may be confused or associated with staphylococcal infection are treated with benzyl penicillin plus flucloxacillin. Macrolides, e.g. azithromycin, can be used in penicillin-allergic patients. Either amoxicillin-clavulanate or modern oral cephalosporins, e.g. cefuroxime, give better results with fewer relapses than penicillin V in acute pharyngo-tonsillitis.

High dose aspirin therapy has a beneficial effect on symptoms and outcome in acute rheumatic fever. Supportive treatment is necessary for cardiac dysfunction. Penicillin should be used for persistent streptococcal infection. To prevent recurrences, daily oral penicillin-V or erythromycin prophylaxis is used. High dose amoxycillin or clindamycin given immediately before dental surgery prevents *Strep. viridans* endocarditis in patients with rheumatic heart disease. Strict fluid and electrolyte balance plus protein restriction are essential in glomerulonephritis.

Prevention

Hospitalized patients should be isolated for 48–72 h, until chemotherapy renders them non-infectious. Eradication of streptococci from the pharynx requires 10 days' therapy. Shorter courses of beta-lactams encourage early relapse.

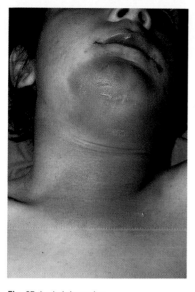

Fig. 87 Ludwig's angina.

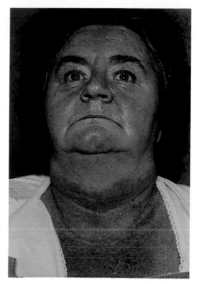

Fig. 88 Ludwig's angina.

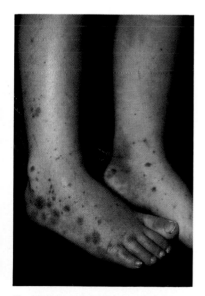

Fig. 89 Henoch–Schönlein purpura.

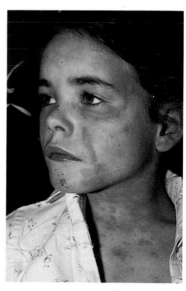

Fig. 90 Erythema marginatum.

17 / Scarlet fever

Aetiology | Beta-haemolytic streptococci of Lancefield's Group A elaborating erythrogenic toxin under the control of a lysogenic bacteriophage.

Incidence | World-wide distribution. Previously common, it is now rarely seen in the developed countries, where it appears a milder disease than formerly.

Pathogenesis | Acquired in the upper respiratory tract via airborne droplet emission from asymptomatic carriers and clinical cases with pharyngeal infections. Wounds may also be a portal of entry. Scarlet fever results from absorption of erythrogenic toxin from the local infective site.

Clinical features | The incubation period of 2–4 days is followed by the sudden onset of sore throat, fever, headache and often vomiting, contrasting with the slower onset of diphtheria and glandular fever. The tonsils are red and flecked with pus, and peritonsillar inflammation and oedema may develop, associated with tender cervical adenitis. The tongue is initially furred and white (Fig. 91) and later smooth and red (Fig. 92). The rash consists of a scarlet blush (Fig. 93) with a punctate erythema, fading on pressure, which spares the circumoral region. It desquamates after a few days, peripheral skin peeling often being most marked on the palms and soles (Fig. 94). Diagnosis is confirmed by a polymorphonuclear leucocytosis, isolation of *Strep. pyogenes* from throat swabs, and rising titres of ASO and anti-DNAase B antibody.

Complications |
- Otitis media
- Local sepsis
- Glomerulonephritis
- Myocarditis with or without rheumatic fever
- Arthralgia affecting small joints

Treatment | Parenteral benzyl penicillin followed by oral amoxycillin (or penicillin V). Erythromycin is substituted in penicillin-allergic patients.

Prevention | Isolation is desirable in the acute phase. Penicillin therapy of contacts may limit institutional outbreaks.

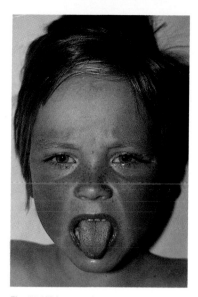

Fig. 91 White strawberry tongue with circumoral pallor.

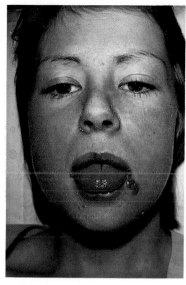

Fig. 92 Red strawberry tongue, perinasal peeling and herpes febrilis.

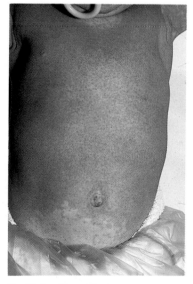

Fig. 93 Punctate erythema.

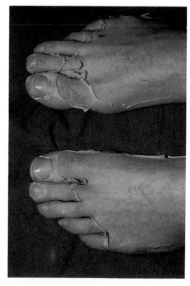

Fig. 94 Peripheral superficial skin peeling.

Aetiology	*Bacillus anthracis*, a Gram-positive sporing bacillus.
Incidence	Rare in UK: more common elsewhere due to enzootic disease.
Pathogenesis	A zoonosis acquired from contact with active cases in sheep, cattle and pigs, and with imported spore-infected hides, hair and bone meal. Spores may be directly inoculated into the skin (cutaneous anthrax), inhaled (pulmonary anthrax) or, more rarely, ingested (intestinal anthrax).
Clinical features	• *Cutaneous anthrax*: a local papule at the site of inoculation is followed by the development of an ulcerated, necrotic eschar (malignant pustule: Figs 95, 96, 97), associated with extensive oedema (Figs 95 & 98), regional adenitis and fever. • *Pulmonary anthrax*: an uncommon, extensive and severe haemorrhagic broncho-pneumonia. • *Intestinal anthrax* (rare in man): varies from mild enteritis to a severe dysentery. • *Bacteraemia*: most commonly follows pulmonary disease. Haemorrhagic meningitis and pleuropericarditis may be associated. Diagnosis is confirmed by the isolation of *B. anthracis* from the malignant pustule, from sputum, stools, blood or CSF as appropriate.
Treatment	Benzyl penicillin (10–20 megaunits/day) for 7 days. Antiserum therapy is no longer used.
Prevention	Notifiable to public health authorities in many countries: strict isolation is necessary. The source must be traced. A vaccine is available for those at risk of occupational exposure, e.g. professional gardeners (bone meal). Potentially infected materials must be rigorously segregated at the port of entry. Strict regulations apply to disposal of infected carcasses.

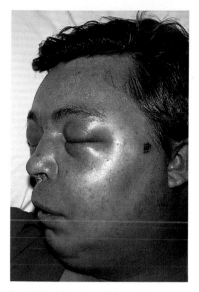

Fig. 95 Facial anthrax with massive oedema (gardener).

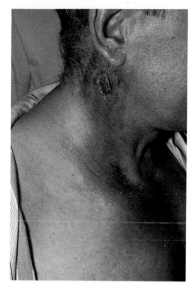

Fig. 96 Cervical eschar (bone meal worker).

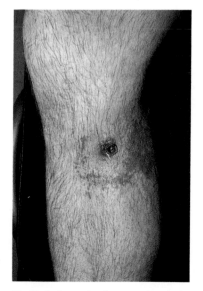

Fig. 97 Eschar on leg (bone meal worker).

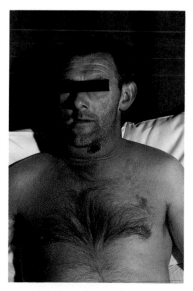

Fig. 98 Eschar and oedema of neck and chest wall (farmer).

19 / Diphtheria

Aetiology	Toxigenic *Corynebacterium diphtheriae*, a Gram-positive bacillus. Toxin production is determined by a lysogenic bacteriophage.
Incidence	World-wide distribution: but rare where there is a high rate of immunization. Travellers to endemic countries (e.g. Eastern Europe/CIS) require active immunization.
Pathogenesis	Airborne droplet transmission from active cases. *C. diphtheriae* multiplies in the upper airways and forms an adherent membrane of bacteria, WBC and necrotic tissue. There is associated oedema of the neck. Laryngeal obstruction can occur in infants. A potent toxin causes later cardiac and neurological complications disrupting protein synthesis and causing demyelination.
Clinical features	The incubation period of 2–4 days is followed by fever, disproportionate tachycardia, malaise, headache and symptoms at the site of invasion: nose, tonsils, pharynx or larynx. Typical adherent membrane appears (Fig. 99), associated with lymphadenopathy and surrounding oedema causing bull-neck appearance (Fig. 100). Stridor may be present in infants with laryngeal diphtheria. Diphtheria toxin causes cardiac dysrhythmias, conduction defects and cardiac failure 1–3 weeks after onset and, later, peripheral neuropathies, including palatal, ocular, diaphragmatic and limb paresis, 3–10 weeks later. Diagnosis is confirmed by isolation of *C. diphtheriae* (Fig. 101) from throat swabs and tests for toxin production.
Treatment	Treatment must not be delayed. IV antitoxin is given if an intradermal test dose shows no significant reaction. Benzyl penicillin or erythromycin are prescribed. Tracheostomy for airway obstruction is rarely necessary today.
Prevention	Notifiable in most countries: strict isolation is mandatory. Toxoid vaccine is given in infancy. Carriers are treated with erythromycin.

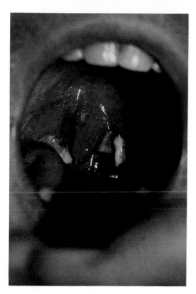

Fig. 99 Pharyngotonsillar diphtheria: note adherent membrane with curled edge.

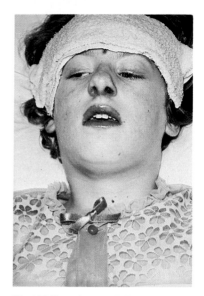

Fig. 100 Nasopharyngeal diphtheria with bloody discharge and bull neck.

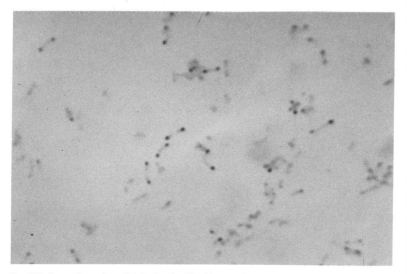

Fig. 101 *Corynebacterium diphtheriae*: bacilli with metachromatic granules.

Aetiology	*Clostridium tetani*, an anaerobic, Gram-positive sporing bacillus, often from manured soil.
Incidence	World-wide distribution: common where there is no immunization, and in rural communities.
Pathogenesis	*Cl. tetani* is an environmental organism which is introduced into deep traumatic anaerobic wounds, including mammalian bites, or into the umbilical stump in neonates. Vegetative multiplication and toxin elaboration follows. Two toxins are produced: • *Tetanolysin*: which causes labile hypertension, dysrhythmias, vasoconstriction and sweating. • *Tetanospasmin*: which fixes to nerves causing muscle spasm.
Clinical features	The incubation period is usually 5–14 days. Muscular spasm and rigidity are invariable and characterized by trismus, risus sardonicus and, later, opisthotonos (Fig. 102). Spasms are triggered by noise, lights or movement. Consciousness and sensation are unimpaired. Respiratory arrest or asphyxia may occur. Neonatal tetanus (Fig. 103) begins 3–10 days after birth and has a very poor prognosis. Tetanus must be differentiated from drug-induced dystonias.
Treatment	Muscular spasms are controlled with intravenous diazepam. Therapeutic paralysis and mechanical ventilation are infrequently required. Human tetanus immunoglobulin and benzyl penicillin are administered.
Prevention	Traumatic wounds must be meticulously cleansed and umbilical stumps kept sterile. Toxoid vaccine should be given to non-immunized or inadequately immunized patients. Human tetanus immunoglobulin is given according to agreed protocols for severe wounds and those over 6 h old. Infants should be routinely immunized. Non-immune mothers can be immunized before delivery. Infection does not confer immunity: immunization is required in convalescence.

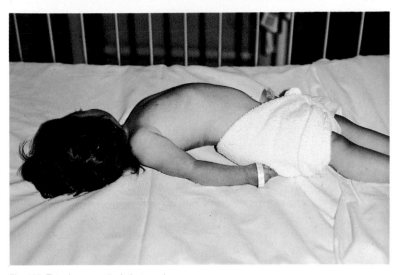

Fig. 102 Tetanic spasm (opisthotonos).

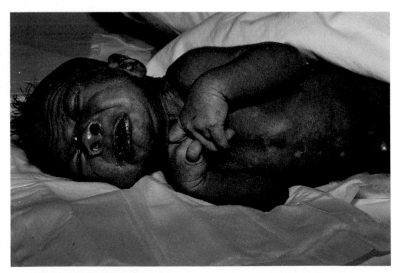

Fig. 103 Neonatal tetanus (wrinkled brow, risus sardonicus and infected umbilical stump).

Aetiology	*Salmonella typhi, Salmonella paratyphi* A and B.
Incidence	World-wide distribution: more common in tropics and with poor sanitation. Faecal contamination of water supplies may cause explosive epidemics.
Pathogenesis	Faecal–oral transmission and contamination of water and food. *S. typhi* not killed by gastric acid, enter the ileum, invade and multiply in the reticulo–endothelial system with subsequent bacteraemia.
Clinical features	The initial bacteraemic phase, lasting about 1 week, is characterized by a step-wise rise in fever, relative bradycardia, constipation, splenomegaly, increasing confusion, dry cough and, less commonly, a pink macular (rose spot) truncal rash (Figs 104 & 105). There follows increasing toxaemia, dehydration, maintained fever, abdominal cramps and diarrhoea (Fig. 106). Recovery commences in the third week but intestinal perforation or haemorrhage may occur. Diagnosis is confirmed by blood and stool cultures, and an '0' antibody response in the Widal test. Long-term stool carriage is rare after quinolone treatment.
Treatment	Fluid and electrolyte balance are strictly monitored. The antibiotics of choice are now quinolones, e.g. ciprofloxacin, orally for 10 days. Cephalosporins are alternatives. Bacterial resistance to other agents is common.
Prevention	Notifiable in most countries: strict isolation is necessary. Good hygiene/sewage disposal and clean water supplies are essential. Polyvalent and monovalent (typhoid alone) intramuscular or subcutaneous vaccines and live attenuated oral typhoid vaccine, which is better tolerated, give partial protection for up to 3 years. Reduction in stool carriage by ciprofloxacin has reduced food and water borne transmission.

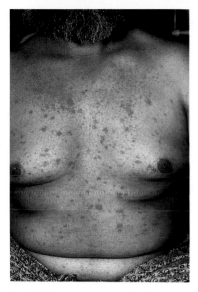

Fig. 104 Extensive 'rose spot' rash in paratyphoid A.

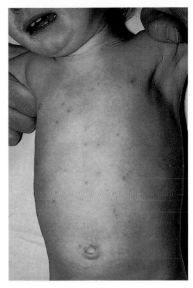

Fig. 105 Rose spots in paratyphoid fever.

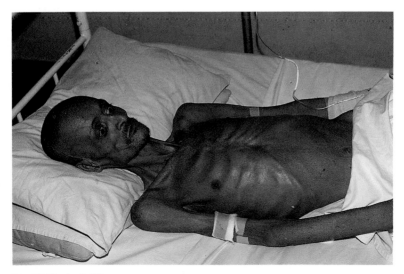

Fig. 106 The 'typhoid' state.

Aetiology	Usually viral. Rotaviruses (see Fig. 111, p. 74) cause 30% of cases together with other small round structured viruses (astroviruses and caliciviruses) and enteroviruses. May also be due to enteropathogenic *Escherichia coli* (EPEC) serotypes (O111, O128, O142, O157 etc.) and *Salmonella*, *Shigella* or *Campylobacter* species. *Cryptosporidium* infection may also be responsible. In at least one-third no aetiological agent is identified.
Incidence	Diarrhoeal illness is amongst the most common causes of morbidity and hospital admission in infants in the UK. It is responsible for up to 25% of infant morbidity in some developing countries and in such areas is the most common cause of death in infancy.
Pathogenesis	Acquisition follows faecal–oral transmission from acute cases (viruses, shigellosis, EPEC), via foodstuffs or milk/water (salmonellosis, campylobacteriosis) or from carriers (salmonellosis). *Cryptosporidium* may spread via water or from animals. Enteritis is caused by either gut wall invasion and inflammation (e.g. shigellosis and salmonellosis), adherence and cytotoxicity (e.g. rotavirus and EPEC enteritis), or invasion of the gut wall plus enterotoxin production (e.g. campylobacteriosis).
Clinical features	The cardinal features are diarrhoea and vomiting, which vary from trivial to profuse. Blood staining of faeces is more typical of invasive disease due to bacteria, especially shigellosis and campylobacteriosis. Fluid loss may cause dehydration, hypovolaemia and hypotension (Figs 107, 108, 109). The anterior fontanelle and eyes appear sunken, skin turgor is decreased, the mucosae are dry and, after initial irritability, there follows apathy and coma. Weight is lost rapidly. Excoriation of the buttocks and perineum may occur (Fig. 110). Bacteraemia may accompany salmonellosis and EPEC enteritis. ➡

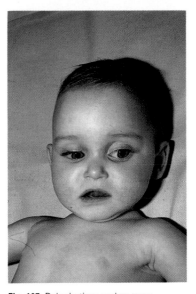

Fig. 107 Dehydration: sunken eyes, corrugated axillary folds and dry mouth.

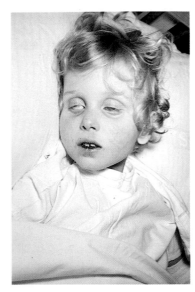

Fig. 108 Severe dehydration.

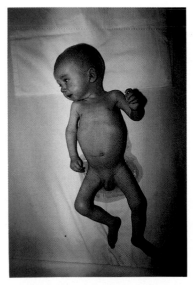

Fig. 109 Dehydrated infant: clear fluid stool after glucose/electrolyte feed.

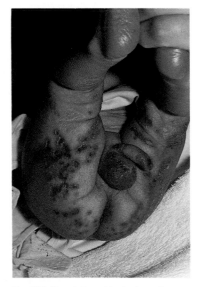

Fig. 110 Excoriation of buttocks and perineum.

Esch. coli 0157 is associated with verotoxin production and may cause severe bloody diarrhoea, complicated by the haemolytic-uraemic syndrome in children and haemorrhagic colitis in adults.

Bacteraemia may accompany salmonellosis and EPEC infection but is uncommon with other bacterial diarrhoeas in Europe and USA. Diagnosis requires stool and, where relevant, blood cultures. Enteropathogenic viruses in stools may be demonstrated by electron microscopy (Fig. 111) or polyacrilamide gel electrophoresis.

Complications

- *Hypernatraemia*: most commonly associated with the use of hypertonic milk feeds (no longer marketed) in early disease, causing, in severe cases, intracranial sinus thrombosis, cerebral oedema with convulsions and neurological defects, and renal damage (Fig. 112).
- *Acute colitis*: a syndrome similar to ulcerative colitis can follow salmonellosis or campylobacteriosis but is usually self-limiting.
- *Lactose intolerance*: Transient disaccharidase deficiency may complicate virus (usually rotavirus) enteritis, and causes persistent diarrhoea. Settling spontaneously within 4–8 weeks, it requires the temporary substitution of non-lactose containing milks.
- *Haemolytic–uraemic syndrome* (*Esch. coli 0157*) may cause microangiopathic anaemia, thrombocytopenia and renal failure.

Treatment

Rehydration using oral or parenteral glucose-electrolyte solutions. Breast-feeding should continue where possible. Antibiotics are usually contraindicated except in bacteraemic infants. Haemolytic uraemic syndrome may require transfusion and dialysis.

Prevention

Many forms notifiable in various countries (e.g. salmonellosis). Hospitalized cases must be isolated. Preventative measures include food and milk hygiene, adequate cooking, e.g. poultry, encouragement of breast-feeding and the provision of clean water supplies and effective sanitation. Rotavirus vaccines are in development.

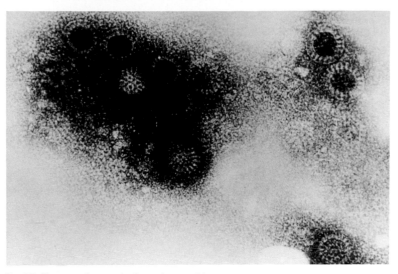

Fig. 111 Electron micrograph of rotavirus particles.

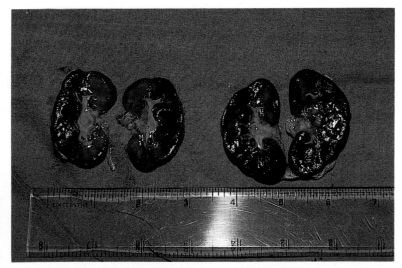

Fig. 112 Bilateral renal thrombosis in dehydrated neonate.

23 / Pseudomembranous colitis

Aetiology	*Clostridium difficile*, a toxin-producing Gram-positive sporing anaerobe.
Incidence	Uncommon, but may occur in sub-epidemic form in surgical wards and where broad spectrum antibiotics are extensively and repeatedly used. It may present during or up to 6 weeks after treatment. Rare spontaneous cases occur.
Pathogenesis	Colonic overgrowth of *Cl. difficile*, induced by antibiotic exposure, is followed by enterotoxin production and mucosal damage typified by summit lesions on colonic mucosa (Fig. 113), glandular disruption, epithelial necrosis and focal inflammation. Macroscopic colonic pseudomembranes are present (Fig. 114). Pseudomembranous colitis most commonly follows broad spectrum antibiotic exposure, e.g. amoxicillin and either parenteral cephalosporins significantly excreted by the biliary route or oral derivatives with poor absorption, both delivering high concentrations to the bowel. It is classically associated with clindamycin. The source of *Cl. difficile* in institutional outbreaks may be related to hospital cross-infection.
Clinical features	• *Mild*: causing slight persistent diarrhoea, self-limiting within 2 weeks in 80%. • *Severe*: frequent bloody diarrhoea with abdominal pain and tenesmus with fever and dehydration. It may progress to toxic dilatation of the colon (Fig. 115), perforation and death. Diagnosis is substantiated by sigmoidoscopy, rectal biopsy and examination of stools for *Cl. difficile* and enterotoxin.
Treatment	Response to oral vancomycin is usually rapid but 10% of patients relapse. Metronidazole is an alternative.
Prevention	Not notifiable: known cases must be isolated to prevent cross colonization of other patients. Non-disposable instruments used rectally should be sterilized with sporicidal disinfectants.

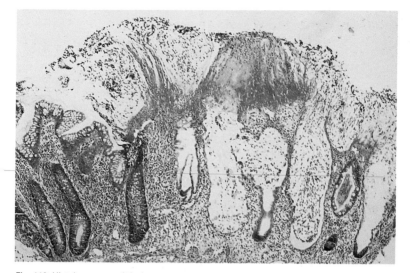

Fig. 113 Histology: summit lesion.

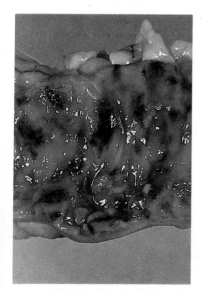

Fig. 114 Colonic pseudomembranes.

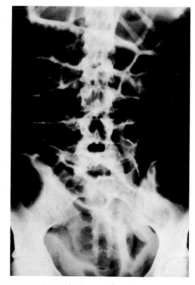

Fig. 115 Toxic dilatation of colon (precolectomy).

Aetiology

Neisseria meningitidis: a Gram-negative diplococcus. Epidemics are usually due to types A, B and C. Other serotypes cause sporadic cases.

Incidence

Epidemic fluctuation: about 1000 sporadic cases per year in the UK, but with local outbreaks. A world-wide pandemic spreading from Asia is currently causing major problems in sub-Saharan Africa. Secondary cases may occur after exposure of close family and nursery school contacts to the index.

Pathogenesis

Spread occurs via airborne droplet transmission from nasopharynx of cases and carriers. Between 10–25% of the healthy population are nasopharyngeal carriers of *N. meningitidis*. Acquisition by a susceptible individual is followed by fulminating bacteraemia with or without meningitis. Others appear to acquire asymptomatic nasopharyngeal carriage. In acute cases, endotoxin release by viable *N. meningitidis* causes massive TNF and interleukin response with antibody-independent complement activation resulting in shock, disseminated intravascular coagulation and generalized Schwartzman reaction (capillary damage, thrombosis and haemorrhage into skin and adrenals). In survivors, immune complex deposition disease may cause arthritis.

Clinical features

- *Fulminating meningococcaemia*: petechiae and ecchymoses (Figs 116–119) are followed by overwhelming shock (see Fig. 120, p. 80), adrenal infarction (see Fig. 121, p. 80) and death from Waterhouse–Friderichsen syndrome (see Fig. 122, p. 80) within 6–18 h of onset. Most common in infants.
- *Bacterial meningitis*: severe toxaemia, meningeal irritation and petechial rash (not always present) associated with a polymorphonuclear CSF pleocytosis plus low CSF sugar and elevated protein. Usually fatal within 24–72 h if untreated. More common in older children and young adults. ➡

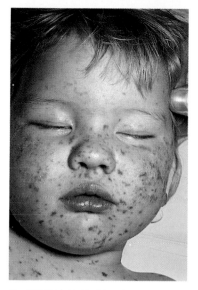

Fig. 116 Petechial facial rash.

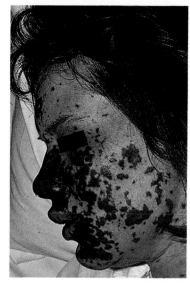

Fig. 117 Ecchymotic facial rash (late stage).

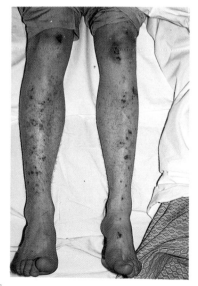

Fig. 118 Haemorrhagic rash (adult with meningitis).

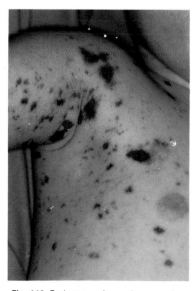

Fig. 119 Ecchymoses in meningococcal septicaemia.

- *Recurrent meningitis*: associated with antibody and complement deficiencies.
- *Pneumonia*: uncommon.
  Diagnosis is established by Gram-stain of *N. meningitidis* in CSF, isolation from CSF and blood cultures, or by detection of antigens in CSF.

Complications

- *Immune complex disease*: arthritis and pericarditis can arise 1 week or more after onset.
- *Skin necrosis*: may follow ecchymotic haemorrhage.
- *Renal tubular damage*: a late phenomenon in those surviving severe disease.

Treatment

Intravenous benzyl penicillin for 5 days. Intrathecal therapy is unnecessary and potentially dangerous. IV ceftriaxone is an alternative. Chloramphenicol should be used for beta-lactam-allergic patients. Steroids, except in massive doses for Waterhouse–Friderichsen syndrome, are of little benefit. Monoclonal antibodies against endotoxin and tumour necrosis factor may prove of benefit in the future.

Prevention

Notifiable in most countries: strict isolation is necessary, but secondary cases amongst hospital contacts are extremely rare.

- *Chemoprophylaxis*: family and nursery school contacts should receive rifampicin plus, in adults, minocycline, for 2 days. Secondary cases mostly occur within 24 h of the index case: chemoprophylaxis should therefore be started immediately. Oral ciprofloxacin (single-dose, used alone) is an alternative. Meningococci persist in the nasopharynx after penicillin treatment and convalescent patients should receive chemoprophylaxis (as above) to protect subsequent contacts.
- *Immunoprophylaxis*: several polysaccharide vaccines are available for types A and C and are becoming generally used, either for control of epidemics, e.g. recent outbreaks in West Africa and at the Haj in Mecca, or individual protection of contacts (together with chemoprophylaxis as above). Type B vaccines are in development.

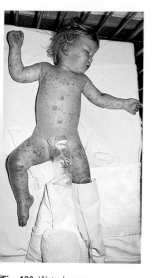

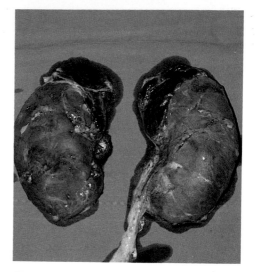

Fig. 120 Waterhouse–Friderichsen syndrome.

Fig. 121 Bilateral haemorrhagic adrenal infarction.

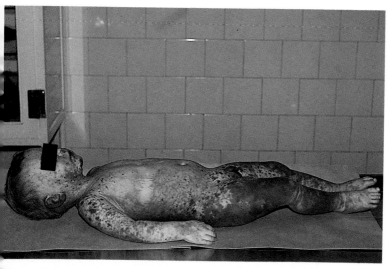

Fig. 122 Death from Waterhouse–Friderichsen syndrome.

25 / Bacterial meningitis (non-meningococcal)

Aetiology	*Streptococcus pneumoniae.* Pittman type B *H. influenzae* (HIB) now rare due to widespread vaccination. Group B streptococci, *Esch. coli* and *Listeria monocytogenes* in infancy.
Incidence	2000 cases/year in the UK.
Pathogenesis	*Strep. pneumoniae*: usually endogenous, invading meninges via blood stream, sinuses, middle ear infections or basal fractures. HIB—an exogenous infection acquired from carriers. Acute inflammatory infiltration of meninges and ventricles is associated with fulminating bacteraemia.
Clinical features	A severe, acute onset illness, characterized within 24–48 h by high fever, headache, neck stiffness (Fig. 123), photophobia, plus vomiting and confusion. Focal CNS signs and coma indicate a poor prognosis. Diagnosis is established by CSF examination (polymorph pleocytosis, low sugar) and detection by Gram-stain, culture or immunological means, e.g. antigen demonstration, of the pathogen in CSF and blood. CSF sampling contraindicated with focal signs or raised intracranial pressure. Consider CT scanning but do not delay treatment.
Complications	<ul><li>Persistent fever: often due to antibiotic therapy.</li><li>Intracranial abscess (rare).</li><li>Sterile subdural effusions (rare).</li><li>CNS abnormalities: decerebrate rigidity (Fig. 124), hydrocephalus, deafness, epilepsy.</li><li>Septic arthritis (pneumococcal disease).</li></ul>
Treatment	IV ceftriaxone is the agent of choice. Vancomycin is added if pneumococcal penicillin resistance is locally prevalent (or confirmed after culture). Amoxycillin is added for listeriosis. Group B streptococcal disease is treated with ampicillin and gentamicin.
Prevention	Notifiable in most countries. Conjugate HIB vaccines are now administered routinely in infancy.

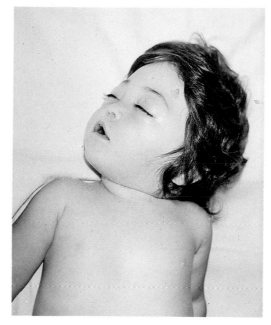

Fig. 123 Neck retraction (severe rigidity).

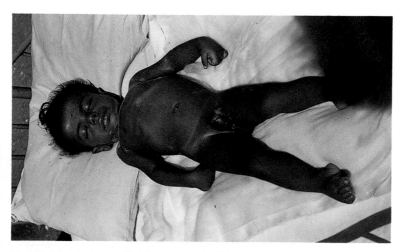

Fig. 124 Decerebrate state (*H. influenzae meningitis*).

Aetiology	Enteroviruses (echo, Coxsackie, and polio viruses), mumps virus, Herpes simplex viruses-1/2.
Incidence	Epidemic fluctuations in incidence, enteroviruses in most summers and, before routine immunization was introduced, mumps every 3–4 years.
Pathogenesis	Enteroviruses spread via faecal–oral route, mostly in children who transmit infection to older family contacts. Mumps spreads by airborne droplet transmission from active cases. Both cause lymphocytic meningitis with minimal brain and spinal parenchymal inflammation.
Clinical features	• *Enteroviruses*: cause a biphasic illness, initially mild prodromal febrile URTI or enteritis followed by recrudescent fever, positional headache, neck and spinal rigidity (Fig. 125), photophobia, vomiting and, in some, a maculopapular rash (Fig. 126) and pharyngitis or conjunctivitis. The patient is usually not very ill.
	• *Mumps meningitis*: causes similar signs of meningeal irritation, usually preceded by salivary gland involvement.
Diagnosis	Lumbar puncture reveals lymphocytic CSF pleocytosis (often particularly high in mumps), normal protein and sugar (may be low in mumps). CSF virus detection by PCR is becoming available. Serology reveals rising titres to causative viruses.
Complications	Echo and Coxsackie viruses rarely cause ascending paralysis similar to poliomyelitis. In adults mumps may be complicated by orchitis, oophoritis, pancreatitis or arthritis.
Treatment	Non-specific: analgesia, anti-emetics and bedrest.
Prevention	Poliovirus infections are notifiable: all cases require strict isolation. Poliovaccine is type specific and has no protective effect against other enteroviruses. Mumps vaccine is available alone and as combined MMR vaccine.

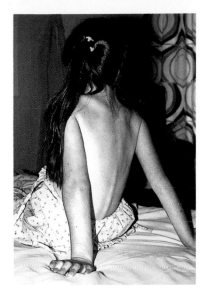

Fig. 125 Tripod sign of spinal rigidity.

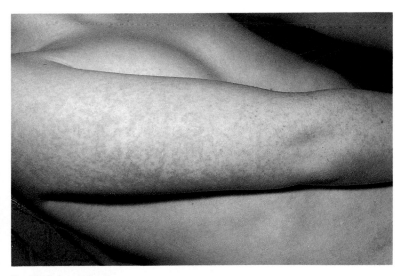

Fig. 126 Enteroviral rash.

27 / Tuberculosis

Aetiology	*Mycobacterium tuberculosis (MTB)* (human and bovine strains).
Incidence	3 million new cases, mostly in children, recognized per year. Rare in the UK, except high risk immigrant groups. Increasing in USA where multiple drug resistance (MDR) is a problem.
Pathogenesis	*Human tuberculosis*: airborne droplet spread from active pulmonary cases, followed by formation of sub-pleural (Ghon) focus and hilar gland involvement (primary complex). Usually heals but may rupture into bronchus, pleura or pulmonary vessels followed by local, pleural, pericardial, bronchial or haematogenous spread. *Bovine tuberculosis*: infected milk may cause tonsillar infection with associated cervical gland caseation and sinuses. Small bowel involvement may cause later tuberculous peritonitis.
Clinical features	**Primary infection** • *Asymptomatic infection with healing*: Skin (Mantoux/Tine) tests become positive in 6–8 weeks: enlarged hilar lymph gland(s) may be obvious on chest X-ray (Fig. 127). Spontaneous healing common but distant sites, e.g. bone, may be seeded with later reactivation. Caseating hilar glands may rupture into contiguous tissue, e.g. pleura. Hypersensitivity phenomena, e.g. erythema nodosum and phlyctenular conjunctivitis are common. • *Tuberculous pleural effusion*: follows rupture of glands into the pleural cavity and can fill the hemithorax (Fig. 128). Tubercle bacilli present in effusion fluid. • *Miliary tuberculosis*: miliary pulmonary infiltration with widespread dissemination plus distant foci including tuberculous meningitis follows bloodstream invasion. Chest X-ray shows 'snowstorm' appearance (Fig. 129). *MTB* cultured from CSF and urine, rarely from blood.

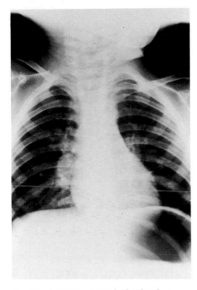

Fig. 127 Primary tuberculosis gland at right hilum.

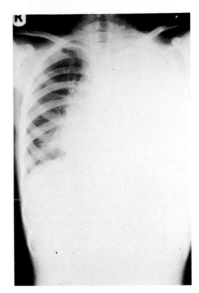

Fig. 128 Primary tuberculous pleural effusion.

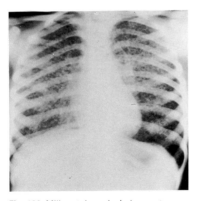

Fig. 129 Miliary tuberculosis (snowstorm appearance).

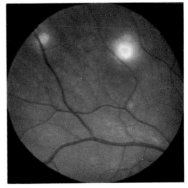

Fig. 130 Choroidal tubercles (TB meningitis) in fundus oculi.

- *Tuberculous meningitis*: insidious onset: drowsiness, headache, confusion for days before signs of meningeal irritation. Choroidal tubercles may be present (see Fig. 130, p. 86). CSF shows lymphocytic pleocytosis, low glucose, high protein and *MTB* on film. Untreated: coma and death invariable within weeks.
- *Tuberculous bronchopneumonia*: either localized to a segment (epituberculosis: Fig. 131) or extensive and bilateral (Fig. 132). Untreated: marked weight loss and death within months.

Late complications
- *Reactivation of pulmonary disease*: in older children and or adults (Fig. 133)
- *Tuberculous pericarditis* (calcification may cause constrictive pericarditis), *osteitis* and *arthritis* (after 5–10 years: Fig. 134), *renal tuberculosis* (after 10–15 years).
- *Tuberculosis and AIDS*: both multiple-drug-resistant *MTB* and *Mycobacterium avium-intracellulare* (MAC) infections are common (Ch. 38).

Treatment

Initial 2-month intensive (3–4 drug) phase of rifampicin plus pyrazinamide (essential to short course therapy) with isoniazid and ethambutol (often omitted in children). Typically followed by 4–6 months consolidation (2 drug) phase using rifampicin and isoniazid. Ill children and those with meningeal and renal disease may require steroid therapy.

Prevention

Notifiable in most countries. Isolation mandatory until treatment renders sputum and urine non-infective (usually 1–2 weeks). Close contacts are screened to detect the source (usually an undiagnosed family member) and other early cases, notably siblings. Those developing positive skin test require chest X-ray. Asymptomatic infections in contacts receive therapy as above (if X-ray abnormal) or isoniazid alone (if X-ray remains normal). BCG vaccination is routinely administered to young teenagers in the UK and is given neonatally in high risk immigrant groups. New immigrants from endemic areas with respiratory symptoms require diagnostic chest X-ray.

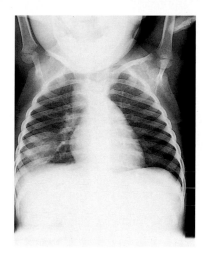

Fig. 131 Epituberculosis in a child.

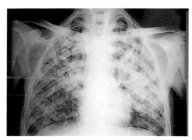

Fig. 132 Tuberculous bronchopneumonia.

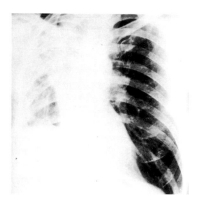

Fig. 133 Adult post-primary pulmonary tuberculosis.

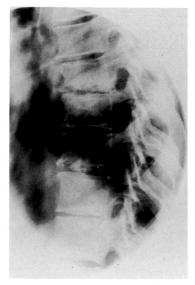

Fig. 134 Tuberculous spondylitis: note erosion of vertebral bodies (Pott's disease).

28 / Pertussis (whooping cough)

Aetiology	*Bordetella pertussis*, a Gram-negative bacillus.
Incidence	Sporadic disease with epidemics every 3–5 years. Decreasing with vaccine uptake but still prevalent in young children.
Pathogenesis	Airborne droplet transmission from active cases. Inflammatory bronchitis is accompanied by mucosal necrosis and mucus hypersecretion, peribronchial infiltration and, in many cases, plugging of airways and absorption collapse. Aspirated pharyngeal commensals cause secondary bacterial bronchitis, pneumonia, abscess formation and segmental collapse.
Clinical features	Incubation period (5–10 days) is followed by upper respiratory catarrh for up to a week. Paroxysmal cough develops, with inspiratory whoop which persists for several weeks. Cough may cause cyanosis, vomiting and apnoea. Chest examination is normal between paroxysms. Diagnosis confirmed by culture of nasopharyngeal swabs and by serology. Peripheral blood demonstrates lymphocytosis.
Complications	• *Respiratory*: secondary bacterial pneumonia, lung abscess and pulmonary collapse (Figs 135 & 136). Common in infancy. Bronchiectasis may follow. • *Neurological*: rare and characterized by convulsions, coma and CNS signs. • *Cough-related*: subconjunctival haemorrhage (Fig. 137), skin petechiae, herniae, rectal prolapse and ulceration of the frenum of the tongue.
Treatment	Erythromycin within 1 week of onset attenuates severity. Secondary bronchopneumonia is treated with a macrolide or amoxycillin.
Prevention	Notifiable: isolate hospitalized cases. Polyvalent vaccine gives 95% protection but may rarely cause encephalopathy. Newer cell constituent vaccines are safer. Erythromycin within 5 days of contact may prevent disease.

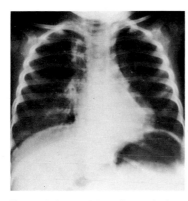

Fig. 135 Left lower lobe collapse: shadow behind the heart.

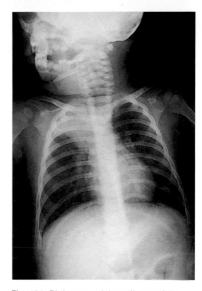

Fig. 136 Right upper lobe collapse: right apex.

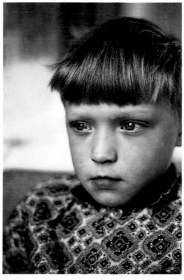

Fig. 137 Subconjunctival haemorrhage.

29 / Acute croup and bronchiolitis

Aetiology	Parainfluenza viruses (75% of croup) and respiratory syncitial virus (RSV) (typically 70% of bronchiolitis).
Incidence	Acute croup usually affects children from 3–36 months: bronchiolitis, infants less than 3 months. Both are cold weather illnesses which are distributed world-wide. Recurrences are common.
Pathogenesis	Spreads by airborne droplet from active cases. In croup, oedema and inflammatory narrowing of upper airways result in stridor and hoarseness. Bronchiolitis is associated with paralysis of cilia, mucus plugging of terminal airways and mucosal necrosis. Secondary infection by pharyngeal commensals may cause bronchopneumonia.
Clinical features	• *Croup*: coryzal syndrome, followed by barking cough, hoarseness, *inspiratory stridor* and respiratory distress, worse at night. Diagnosed by tissue culture and serology. • *Bronchiolitis*: often afebrile, the infant is distressed with intercostal recession, nasal flare, tracheal tug, cough, crepitations and rhonchi. Dyspnoea interrupts feeding, causing dehydration. RSV demonstrable in mucus by immunofluorescence microscopy or tissue culture. • *Chest X-ray*: may show either peribronchitis (Fig. 138) or bronchopneumonia.
Treatment	Severely ill cases are treated with oxygen-enriched, humidified air. Severe croup requires use of IV hydrocortisone to clear the oedematous airway: tracheostomy is rarely necessary. Babies with bronchiolitis may need antibiotics (such as erythromycin), bronchodilators, IV fluids and hydrocortisone in severe cases. Aerosolised ribavirin is useful for severe RSV infection in immunosuppressed children.
Prevention	Active cases are highly infectious and should be isolated from other young children. RSV vaccines are under development but not generally available.

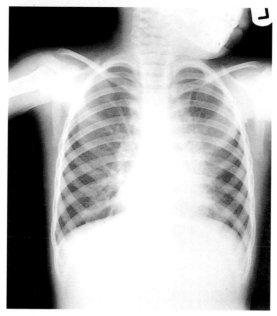

Fig. 138 Diffuse peribronchial infiltration.

Aetiology

Community acquired pneumonia (CAP) may be caused by *Strep. pneumoniae* (>50% of cases), by other bacteria or by atypical pathogens, which may account for 20–30% of cases. *Atypical pneumonia* is most frequently caused by *Mycoplasma pneumoniae* and *Chlamydia pneumoniae.* Q fever (*Coxiella burneti*), psittacosis-ornithosis (*Chl. psittaci*) and Legionnaires' disease (Ch. 31) are less common causes. *Lobar pneumonia* (Fig. 139) affecting a single segment or lobe of the lung is classically caused by *Strep. pneumoniae* and *bronchopneumonia* (Fig. 140), involving multiple sites, by atypical pathogens, *Staph. aureus*, and *H. influenzae*, the latter most frequently in children and chronic bronchitics. Diffuse, often bilateral, hazy infiltration on chest X-ray is likely to be either atypical or viral.

Incidence

Usually sporadic but atypical infection shows epidemic variation. Thus, *Mycoplasma pneumoniae* infection has 3–4 year cycles, incidence rising towards the winter. Psittacosis affects many birds including parrots and budgerigars, pigeons and game birds. In man, it usually follows accidental contact with reactivation of latent infection in birds, usually due to stress, e.g. overcrowding in aviaries, and is seen in fanciers and handlers. Pregnant women are very susceptible to ovine chlamydial disease (and should avoid lambing). Q-fever is a disease of sheep, goats and cattle, ocasionally also seen in vets and farmers.

   Severe pneumococcal disease occurs in cirrhotics, alcoholics and in patients with immunodeficiency, e.g. post-splenectomy, AIDS and sickle cell anaemia. *Staphylococcal* infections may complicate influenza, other viral URTI and intubation in the ICU. *Community-acquired Gram-negative pneumonia* is rare but may be seen in alcoholics, inmates of community care facilities for the elderly and the immunodeficient, particularly in granulocytopenic cancer patients. *Aspiration*

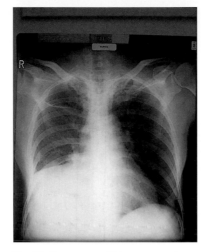

Fig. 139 Pneumococcal lobar pneumonia.

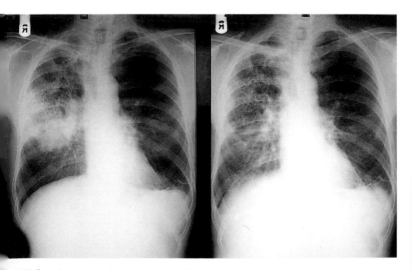

Fig. 140 Bronchopneumonia at onset and during convalescence.

cancer patients. *Aspiration pneumonia*, involving oro-pharyngeal anaerobes, may occur in neurologically-impaired or unconscious patients.

Epidemiology and pathogenesis

Classical pneumococcal lobar pneumonia follows inhalation of naso-pharyngeal commensals which initiate a focus of infection within the lung and result in acute inflammation, consolidation (Fig. 141) and potential complications including local and bacteraemic spread.

Atypical organisms are inhaled via droplet emission from active cases (mycoplasma pneumonia) or exposure to aerosols/dust in contaminated environments (psittacosis, Q fever). They are either intracellular or cell surface associated (Mycoplasma) pathogens. Low grade inflammation results in widespread pneumonitis.

Clinical features

- *Epidemiological aspects*: a history of previous illness, drug exposure, travel history (Legionnaires' disease), animal contact (Q fever) or bird contact (psittacosis), or contact with a patient (viral pneumonias) may be relevant.
- *Prodromal phase*: pneumococcal pneumonia has a sudden onset, often without preceding illness. Atypical pneumonias have incubation periods of 1–3 weeks and are often preceded by a systemic prodrome lasting for up to a week, with pyrexia, sore throat, myalgia and arthralgia.
- *Uncomplicated atypical pneumonia*: is associated with dry cough and a mild pneumonitis which can be patchy, multifocal or perihilar. These changes may only be detectable by X-ray (Fig. 142), clinical signs of consolidation often being absent. Pleurisy is uncommon and haemoptysis is rare. The illness may last for 2–3 weeks. Severe infections may occur but mortality is less than 3%.
- *Uncomplicated pneumococcal disease*: presents with rapid onset and signs of localized consolidation and systemic toxaemia, with rigors/pyrexia. Pleural pain, e.g. during coughing and deep breathing, is common and haemoptysis may occur.➡

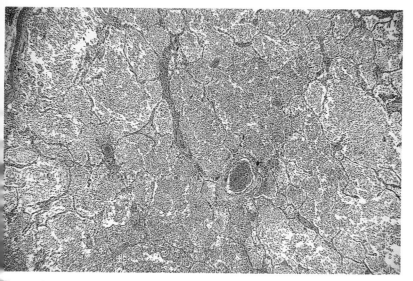

Fig. 141 Consolidation in pneumonia: histopathology.

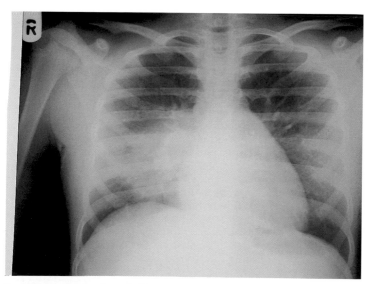

Fig. 142 X-ray changes in atypical (*mycoplasma*) pneumonia.

- *Severe CAP*: usually but not exclusively due to bacterial pathogens. Characterized by hyperventilation (RR > 30/min), arterial hypoxia (pO2 < 8.5 kPa), hypotension (diastolic pressure <60 mm/Hg), mental confusion, multilobar involvement, secondary renal and hepatic dysfunction. Bacteraemia is often present in pneumococcal disease, in which mortality may exceed 30%.

Diagnosis

Chest X-ray demonstrates lobar consolidation or multifocal opacification (Figs 139–144). Bacterial pathogens can be isolated from sputum, blood and tissue cultures. Pneumococcal antigen is present in sputum and urine. Serology is required to confirm atypical infection: PCR is being developed for *M. pneumoniae* infection.

Complications

- *Pneumococcal pneumonia*: lung abscess, empyema, bacteraemia and, in untreated disease, metastatic infection including meningitis, endocarditis and septic arthritis.
- *Mycoplasma pneumoniae pneumonia*: arthritis, haemolytic anaemia, encephalitis and Stevens–Johnson syndrome (Ch. 34).
- *Q fever*: endocarditis and hepatic involvement (likely if phase I antibody persists).
- *Psittacosis-ornithosis*: renal failure, encephalitis, endocarditis and DIC.

Treatment

- *General principles*: differentiation of pneumococcal from atypical pneumonias can be difficult. In the latter, patients tend to be younger, to have been ill for longer, to have had a prodromal illness and, often, to have failed to respond to empirical penicillin therapy. However, these features are not diagnostic and infections with more than one pathogen may also occur. Therefore, in severe disease, combination therapy is required. Benzyl penicillin or amoxicillin (oral) are the drugs of choice for pneumococcal infection *in the lung*. Macrolides, which reach the intracellular habitat, are required for atypical infection and Legionnaires' disease. Regimes incorporating amoxicillin (or co-amoxiclav) plus either clarithromycin or erythromycin provide broad spectrum cover.

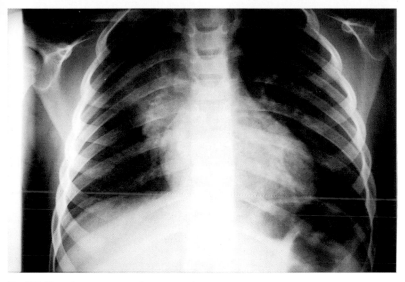

Fig. 143 *Mycoplasma pneumoniae* pneumonia.

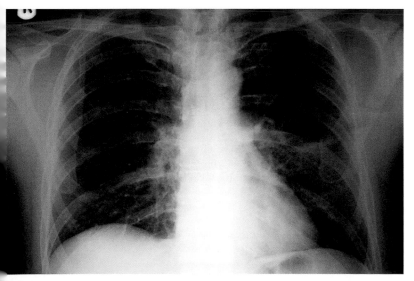

Fig. 144 Psittacosis pneumonia.

- *Bacterial resistance*: intermediate penicillin/amoxicillin resistance in pneumococci and *H. influenzae* has reached 20–40% in many parts of the world. Many of these strains are also erythromycin resistant.
- *Pneumococcal pneumonia*: high-dose benzyl penicillin or amoxicillin are effective for pneumonia caused by sensitive or intermediately sensitive isolates alike. Cefotaxime or ceftriaxone must be used if systemic spread has occurred. Vancomycin is mandatory if meningitis is suspected and may be required for pneumonia if high-level (mic >2 mg/l) penicillin resistant pneumococci increase in prevalence. New fluoroquinolones, e.g. trovafloxacin/grepafloxacin, are promising alternatives.
- *Staphylococcal pneumonia*: combinations, e.g. flucloxacillin plus fusidic acid, are superior to monotherapy.
- *Gram-negative pneumonia*: either ciprofloxacin or imipenem are effective. Both are used if *P. aeruginosa* infection is suspected.
- *Atypical pneumonia*: erythromycin, clarithromycin (IV-oral) or azithromycin (3 day oral course) are preferred for *Mycoplasma* and *Chl. pneumoniae* infections. Tetracycline is recommended for Q fever and psittacosis.
- *Treatment guidelines*: recommendations formulated by the British Thoracic Society (under revision) are summarized in Table 1.

Prevention

Polyvalent pneumococcal vaccine is available for predisposed patients, e.g. sickle cell disease, post-splenectomy and severe bronchitis. Mycoplasma and human chlamydial respiratory infections are not preventable except by avoidance of affected subjects in epidemics.

Psittacosis and Q fever require avoidance of exposure and hygiene measures in bird and animal husbandry, respectively. Experimental vaccines are not generally applicable. Routine isolation of active cases is not necessary.

Table 1. British Guidelines: Antibiotic management of community acquired pneumonia in adults admitted to hospital

Pneumonia syndrome	Recommended antibiotic therapy
Uncomplicated pneumonia without mortality risk factors	Oral amoxicillin, or IV benzyl penicillin or ampicillin, or erythromycin for penicillin-allergic patients
Severe pneumonia of uncertain aetiology	Erythromycin (high dose), plus cephalosporin, e.g. cefotaxime or ceftriaxone
Staphylococcal pneumonia	Flucloxacillin (addition of fusidic acid or gentamicin may be advantageous)
Legionnaires' disease (LD) and Mycoplasma pneumoniae pneumonia	Erythromycin (high dose), plus rifampicin or ciprofloxacin for severe LD.
Q fever and Psittacosis	Tetracycline
Aspiration pneumonia (e.g. unconscious patient)	Amoxicillin plus metronidazole or clindamycin

(British Thoracic Society: British Journal of Hospital Medicine 1993;49:346–350)

31 / Legionnaires' disease

Aetiology | *Legionella pneumophila* and related species: small Gram-negative cocco-bacilli.

Incidence | Account for 3–5% of atypical pneumonias. Sporadic incidence mixed with common source outbreaks (hotels and hospitals). Frequent nosocomial pathogen in immunosuppressed patients.

Pathogenesis | Legionellae are omnipresent in warm water environments, e.g. air-conditioning condensers, shower systems, cooling towers, from which inhalation of aerosols causes sporadic cases or point source outbreaks. Multisystem involvement follows, with pneumonitis, renal failure and cerebellar encephalopathy.

Clinical features | The incubation period of 2–10 days is followed by a non-specific syndrome of fever, malaise, myalgia, rigors, headache and diarrhoea. Confusion is prominent. Beta-lactam therapy typically fails. Dry cough develops but respiratory signs are minimal initially: crepitations, often multifocal, develop days later. Consolidation is usually absent. Chest X-ray shows lobar, multifocal or diffuse infiltration (Figs 145 & 146): an effusion may be present. Early diagnosis is achieved by detection of antigen in urine or bronchial/lung biopsy, and confirmed by serology (IFAT). Untreated disease lasts 2–3 weeks.

Complications | Renal and respiratory failure, and cerebellar ataxia may occur. The mortality may exceed 25% falling to <10% with effective therapy.

Treatment | IV erythromycin is the current drug of choice but clarithromycin and azithromycin are more effective in animal models. Rifampicin or ciprofloxacin are added for severely ill patients.

Prevention | Case-to-case transmission does not occur: isolation is not necessary. Infected water systems, especially in hospitals, should be adequately chlorinated. Notification required in some countries.

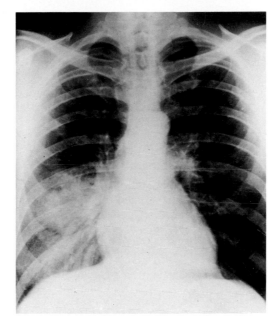

Fig. 145 Legionnaires' pneumonitis.

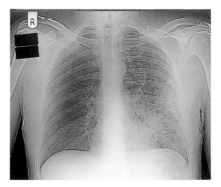

Fig. 146 Legionnaires' pneumonitis.

Aetiology	*Strep. pneumoniae* (post-pneumonic), *Staph. aureus* (post-pneumonic), mixed oropharyngeal anaerobes, e.g. *Bacteroides* and *Prevotella* spp. (post-aspiration), mixed flora (post-embolic abscess).
Incidence	A sporadic endogenous infection.
Pathogenesis	May complicate primary pneumonia (pneumococci, staphylococci and Gram-negative bacilli), lobar collapse, aspiration of oral secretions (alcoholic, epileptic, comatose or ventilated patients), pulmonary infarction and tricuspid endocarditis (usually *Staph. aureus* in IV drug misusers).
Clinical features	• *Presents as*: either a complication of pneumonia, unexplained fever in comatose or ventilated patients, recurrence of fever after pulmonary embolism or tricuspid endocarditis, haemoptysis or pyrexia of unknown origin. • *Physical signs*: can be minimal in the absence of overlying pleurisy or complicating empyema. Foul sputum usually indicates anaerobic infection. Blood and sputum cultures are mandatory. • *Chest X-ray*: either shows a rounded opacity with an air-fluid level (Fig. 147), multiple opacities or cavitation within an area of consolidation.
Treatment	Prolonged antibiotic courses of 6–8 weeks are usually required. Post-pneumonic and aspiration abscesses should be treated with benzyl penicillin plus metronidazole (or clindamycin). Staphylococcal lung abscesses require cloxacillin plus fusidic acid or clindamycin. Complicating empyema must be repeatedly aspirated to dryness or surgically drained.
Prevention	Important factors include adequate therapy of primary pneumonias, physiotherapy and tracheostomy care of comatose or ventilated patients, and rapid bronchoscopic clearance of obstructed airways.

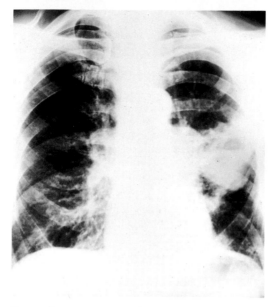

Fig. 147 Post-aspiration lung abscess: fluid level.

Aetiology	Multiple precipitants: usually drugs, notably the combined contraceptive pill and sulphonamides, but including many diseases, particularly streptococcal disease and acute sarcoidosis, plus primary tuberculosis, chronic inflammatory bowel disease and intestinal infections, e.g. yersinosis and campylobacteriosis.
Incidence	Uncommon. Streptococcal infections are the commonest cause in children; acute sarcoidosis and contraceptive pill in young women.
Pathogenesis	A non-infective, non-suppurative localized vasculitis caused by an immunologically mediated reaction to infective or chemical stimuli, or immunologically based disease.
Clinical features	Acutely tender, circumscribed, erythematous skin nodules, 1–4 cm diameter, usually confined to anterior surface of legs below knees (Figs 148 & 149) but sometimes on extensor surfaces of arms. May appear successively for several weeks but usually settle spontaneously within a few weeks if drug or infection related. May persist or recur in sarcoidosis or autoimmune disease. In acute sarcoidosis erythema nodosum is usually associated with arthritis, hilar adenopathy and fever, and occasionally with phlyctenular conjunctivitis and parotitis.
	Diagnosis requires careful enquiry into drug/chemical exposure and identification of infective or inflammatory causes. Serum ACE, Kveim test and Tco are useful for sarcoidosis. Primary TB must be excluded.
Treatment	Removal of the aetiological factor, e.g. cessation of drugs, eradication of infection or treatment of autoimmune disease. If not contraindicated by aetiology (e.g. infections), steroids may have a beneficial effect.
Prevention	May require isolation, dependent on causation. Avoidance of previously recognized drug precipitants.

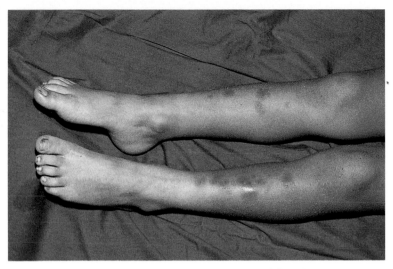

Fig. 148 Early discrete erythema nodosum (due to streptococcal disease).

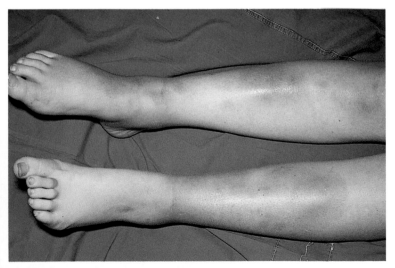

Fig. 149 Late coalescent erythema nodosum (due to sarcoidosis).

Aetiology	May complicate therapy with various drugs including sulphonamides and penicillins, and infections caused by *Mycoplasma pneumoniae*, *Herpes simplex* and streptococci.
Incidence	Sporadic and uncommon.
Pathogenesis	Results from immune hypersensitivity mechanisms of uncertain type which cause vasculitis in the skin, mucous membranes and conjunctivae leading to vesiculo-bullous lesions. Possibly an extension of erythema multiforme in some patients.
Clinical features	Conjunctival, nasal, genital, rectal and mucocutaneous lesions of variable severity. Skin lesions are almost invariably present, commonly on the hands and feet. These commence as a multiform, target-lesion type of eruption (Fig. 150) subsequently progressing to vesiculation and bulla formation (Figs 151 & 152), which may coalesce to an exfoliative picture. Erosive lesions are found on the lips, buccal mucosa, tongue (Fig. 153) and genitalia. Evolution and regression takes place over 2–3 weeks and healing may be accompanied by desquamation, skin pigmentation or superficial scarring. Nowadays rarely fatal, the original descriptions of long acting sulphonamide-induced SJS quoted an infant mortality of 25%.
Complications	Secondary bacterial skin and oral infection is common. Recurrent *Herpes simplex* infections may precipitate further episodes of Stevens–Johnson syndrome.
Treatment	Most cases require symptomatic therapy alone. Secondary skin infections may require treatment with flucloxacillin. Precipitating *M. pneumoniae* infections are treated with erythromycin. Steroids are of unproven benefit despite often being used.
Prevention	None presently available. Aetiologically-related drugs must be avoided.

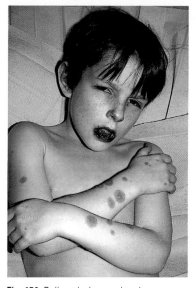

Fig. 150 Bullous lesions and oral ulceration.

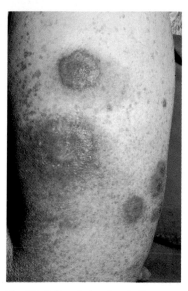

Fig. 151 Bullous lesions (atypical).

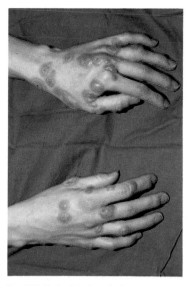

Fig. 152 Vesiculobullous lesions.

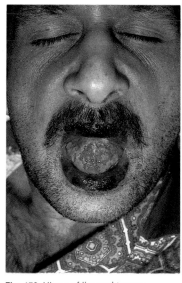

Fig. 153 Ulcers of lips and tongue.

Aetiology

Many antibiotics cause skin rashes, most notably the penicillins, cephalosporins and sulphonamides. Rashes are less commonly caused by erythromycin, chloramphenicol, clindamycin, tetracyclines and quinolones, and only rarely follow the use of aminoglycosides. A maculopapular rash is almost invariable when patients with glandular fever (or lymphoproliferative disorders) receive ampicillin (less common with amoxicillin).

Incidence

The overall incidence is approximately:
- Penicillins: 2–3% (ampicillin up to 7%).
- Cephalosporins: 1–2% (10% of penicillin-allergic patients also react to cephalosporins).
- Sulphonamides: 5% (in AIDS patients receiving co-trimoxazole the incidence may exceed 50%).

Pathogenesis

Antibiotics may engender immediate hypersensitivity (IgE-mediated) reactions, usually causing urticaria, or delayed reactions both of the serum-sickness (IgG-mediated) type and by other ill understood mechanisms, including induction of sensitized lymphocytes. Reactions may relate either to the parent antibiotic, high molecular weight polymers, or to metabolites.

Clinical features

The penicillins, cephalosporins and sulphonamides may all cause urticaria (Fig. 154), morbilliform eruptions (Fig. 155), erythema multiforme (Fig. 156) and Stevens–Johnson syndrome (Ch. 34).

Complications

Usually transient but may be part of a generalized hypersensitivity reaction. Urticaria may presage anaphylaxis if re-exposure occurs.

Treatment

The causative antibiotic must be stopped at once. Early treatment of urticaria with antihistamines (or corticosteroids) may hasten recovery and are also useful for pruritus associated with morbiliform penicillin/cephalosporin rashes. Treatment is otherwise symptomatic.

Prevention

Implicated antibiotics should be avoided.

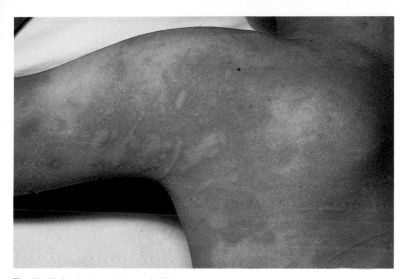

Fig. 154 Urticaria (caused by penicillin).

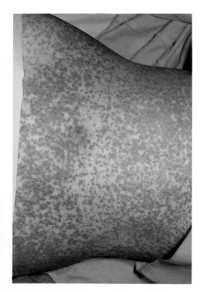

Fig. 155 Morbilliform rash (caused by ampicillin).

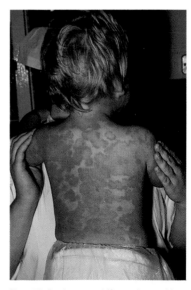

Fig. 156 Erythema multiforme (caused by sulphonamide).

Aetiology	*Treponema pallidum*, a spirochaete.
Incidence	World-wide distribution: high incidence in male homosexuals.
Pathogenesis	Sexually transmitted: man is the only host. The primary chancre appears 9–90 days after sexual contact, followed weeks to months later by the secondary phase. Secondary disease merges into latent endarteritic syphilis in which physical signs are absent but serology, as in secondary syphilis, is positive. Tertiary syphilis causes neurological or cardiovascular disease years later. Both primary and secondary syphilis are highly infectious.
Clinical features	Secondary syphilis mimics many skin infections and infestations, including mononucleosis, acute exanthemata, erythema multiforme, condylomata accuminata, alopecia areata and oral or vaginal candidiasis. Macular, maculopapular, pustular and nodular skin lesions with vesicles last for 1–2 months (Fig. 157). They occur mainly on the palms and soles (Fig. 158). Condylomata are non-tender, moist greyish plaques in intertriginous areas, frequently in the perineum. These and mucosal 'snail track' ulcers are highly infectious. Fever, laryngitis, pharyngitis, arthralgia, painless lymphadenopathy and weight loss occur. The diagnosis of secondary syphilis is confirmed by dark ground examination of exudates for *T. pallidum* and positive serology (TPHA and Elisa for anti-treponemal IgM).
Treatment	Syphilis should always be referred to a specialist physician. In the USA a single dose of 2.4 megaU of benzathine penicillin remains in favour. In the UK, intramuscular procaine penicillin for 10–21 days or intramuscular bicillin may be substituted. Tetracycline in high dose for 28 days may be used for penicillin allergic patients. Herxheimer reactions may be covered with corticosteroids.

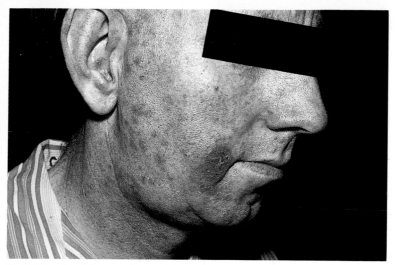

Fig. 157 Papulonodular secondary syphilitic rash.

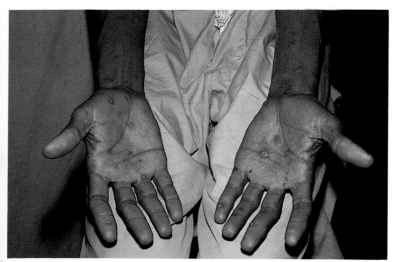

Fig. 158 Palmar lesions in secondary syphilis.

Aetiology	*Neisseria gonorrhoeae*, a Gram-negative diplococcus.
Incidence	A rare, sporadic complication of genital, anorectal and oropharyngeal gonorrhoea.
Pathogenesis	Occurs as a complicating bacteraemia with organ involvement in patients with gonorrhoea.
Clinical features	Initially presents as pyrexia of unknown origin accompanied by sparse, violaceous macular or vesicular skin lesions (Figs 159 & 160), or as a pyrexia with organ involvement, most commonly arthritis (80%). Monarticular septic arthritis usually presents a week or more after onset. Polyarticular, hypersensitivity-mediated small joint arthritis may present within a few days. Endocarditis is an uncommon complication but prior to effective chemotherapy, the gonococcus caused 10% of cases. Diagnosis is by blood culture and isolation of *N. gonorrhoeae* either from endocervical, vaginal, urethral, anorectal and pharyngeal swabs, or from joint fluid. Concomitant syphilis and infection with *Chlamydia trachomatis* should be excluded.
Treatment	• For penicillin-sensitive organisms, a 10 day course of high dose benzyl penicillin is adequate. Septic arthritis or endocarditis should receive 4–6 weeks' treatment. • Penicillinase (beta-lactamase) producing *N. gonorrhoeae* (PPNG) infections receive either oral ciprofloxacin (500 mg, twice daily) or IV ceftriaxone (1 g daily) for 7 days. Single doses of these agents and spectinomyin (2 g) are effective for non-invasive genital and pharyngeal disease. • Coexistent chlamydial urethritis: is treated with either doxycycline (100–200 mg/day) for 7–10 days or a single 1 g dose of azithromycin.
Prevention	Not notifiable: hospitalized cases should be isolated. Routine contact tracing should be undertaken.

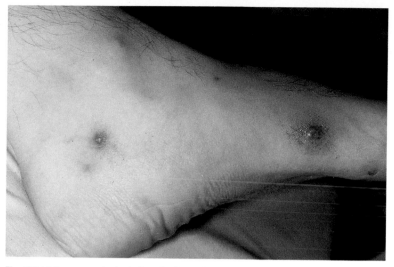

Fig. 159 Violaceous vesicular lesions (iodine self-medication).

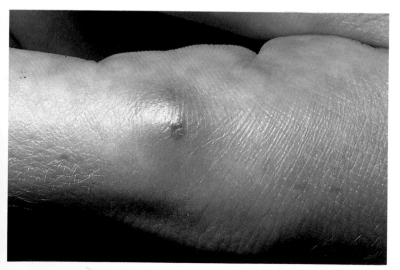

Fig. 160 Papulovesicular lesion.

38 / Acquired immune deficiency syndrome (AIDS)

Aetiology

Human immunodeficiency viruses types 1 and 2 (HIV-1/2), RNA retroviruses which attach to CD4 lymphocytes and CNS cells.

Incidence

World-wide, predominantly caused by HIV-1. By mid-1996 globally, 21 million adults and almost 1 million children had been reported to be infected, 42% of whom are female. Although only 1.5 million have been reported to have developed AIDS, the UN estimates that there have been 7.7 million cases (77% in Africa) with a cumulative mortality of 4.5 million adults and 1.3 million children.

AIDS was originally recognized as a combination of rare diseases, e.g. *Pneumocystis carinii* pneumonitis (Fig. 161) or Kaposi's sarcoma (Figs 162, and 166, 167, p. 120), with acquired immune deficiency in previously healthy homosexual men who were HIV positive. Heterosexual transmission is most important in Africa, where the seroprevalence in young sexually active people may reach 20–40%, but it is increasingly observed in Europe and the USA. IV drug misusers transmit HIV infection via contaminated needles and equipment and also by associated sexual contact/prostitution. Vertical, perinatal and post-natal infection occurs, e.g. after breast-feeding.

Pathogenesis

HIV invades CNS cells leading to cerebral atrophy and AIDS dementia complex. Continuing virus multiplication in CD4 (T4 helper) lymphocytes causes cell mediated immunodeficiency. CD4 counts under $200/mm^3$ correlate with onset of symptomatic illness. The incubation period from infection to development of AIDS is 7–8 years (less in children and those aged >40 years). Almost all HIV infections ultimately result in AIDS.➡

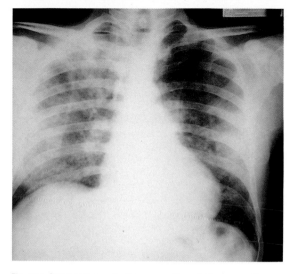

Fig. 161 Chest radiograph: *Pneumocystis carinii* pneumonitis.

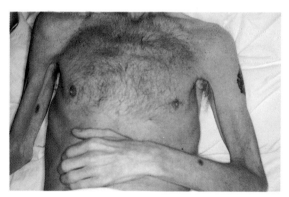

Fig. 162 Cachexia and early Kaposi's sarcoma lesions.

The CDC classification of HIV infection comprises 4 stages. *Stage I* is the acute, glandular fever-like infection after which sero-conversion occurs. *Stage II* refers to asymptomatic infection, leading either via intermediate *Stage III*, Progressive Generalized Lymphadenopathy (PGL) characterized by palpable glands (>1 cm) in two or more non-adjacent sites for >3 months, with or without lassitude, lethargy, sweating, diffuse myalgia and arthralgia, or directly to *Stage IV*:

- *Stage IV A* (AIDS-related complex): constitutional disease plus either fever (>38°C), diarrhoea for >1 month or involuntary weight loss of >10% (see Fig. 162, p. 116).
- *Stage IV B*: CNS disease, myelopathy, neuropathy, dementia or personality change.
- *Stage IV C1*: AIDS defining infections with *Pneumocystis carinii*, cryptococci, toxoplasma, cryptosporidia, and *M. avium-intracellulare* etc.
- *Stage IV C2*: oral hairy leucoplakia, zoster, bacteraemic salmonellosis, tuberculosis, etc.
- *Stage IV D*: malignancies, KS, cerebral and non-Hodgkin's lymphomas.
- *Stage IV E*: chronic lymphoid interstitial pneumonitis (CLIP—normally children), Hodgkin's disease, carcinoma, thrombocytopenia and diseases not otherwise classified.

AIDS commonly presents with PCP: increasing dyspnoea reflecting profound hypoxia which worsens dramatically on exercise. Chest X-ray later shows diffuse opacification. PCP may also present acutely and pneumothorax can occur. The organism is detected in induced sputum, lavage fluid or lung biopsy. Children may present with CLIP. Febrile mycobacterial infection is be detected by blood or bone-marrow culture.

Diarrhoea is commonly due to cryptosporidiosis or salmonellosis but also to HIV infection, CMV colitis and strongyloidiasis. CMV infections, which are common, also cause retinitis (see Fig. 61, p. 42) and pneumonitis. Pure HIV retinitis (Fig. 163) may occur. Oropharygeal and oesophageal candidosis are common (Fig. 164). Oral hairy leucoplakia (see Fig. 165, p. 120) is probably viral in origin.

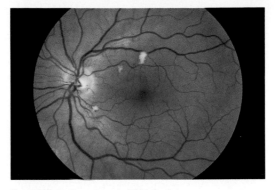

Fig. 163 Retinal exudates in HIV infection.

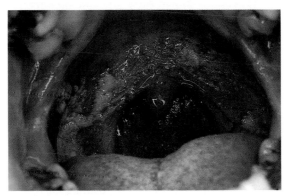

Fig. 164 Oral candidosis.

Male homosexuals often present with Kaposi's sarcoma lesions, typically purple/brown, painless, non-pruritic areas flush with the skin or raised strawberry-like skin plaques (Figs 162, p. 116, Fig. 166). Varying initially, they become persistent, enlarge and coalesce, and may bleed. KS can also affect the lungs and other internal organs in addition to producing skin and oral lesions (Fig. 167).

Fits, dementia and focal CNS signs are usually due either to HIV encephalopathy (see Fig. 168, p. 122), toxoplasma encephalitis (see Fig. 169, p. 122) or lymphoma. CSF examination and CT or MRI scanning are required. Cryptococcal meningitis presents with fever and headache rather than with meningism.

In full blown AIDS, multiple opportunistic infections and tumours may commonly coexist. Diagnosis of one disease does not exclude others as causes of presenting symptoms.

Management

Counselling, support and education as to avoidance of risk factors are vital. HIV antibody-positive individuals should be regularly monitored both clinically and with CD4 counts and estimations of P24 antigen, immunoglobulins and beta-2 microglobulin to assess progression. PCR is used to assess the HIV burden.

Specific therapy includes:

1. *Anti-HIV treatment*: is continuously being revised. Current suggestions for starting therapy are any of the following: CD4 count $<300/mm^3$; plasma viral load $>10\,000-50\,000$ HIV RNA copies/ml or viral load in the range from detectable to 10 000/ml with a falling CD4 count; clinical symptoms irrespective of other parameters. Combinations of two nucleoside analogues, e.g. zidovudine (AZT, ZDV) with didanosine (ddI), zalcitabine (ddC) or lamivudine (3TC) improve CNS symptoms and laboratory parameters, reduce the frequency of opportunistic infection and may lessen the risk of viral resistance. Unacceptable side effects or failure with nucleoside analogue combinations suggests the addition of, or a switch to other combinations including non–nucleoside reverse transcriptase inhibitors or protease inhibitors.

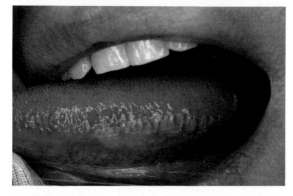

Fig. 165 Oral hairy leucoplakia.

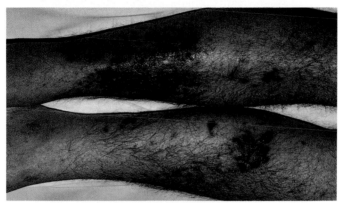

Fig. 166 Extensive Kaposi's sarcoma of the legs.

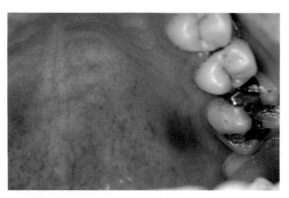

Fig. 167 Kaposi's sarcoma of gums and palate.

2. *Anti-tumour therapy*: local radiotherapy, vincristine, vinblastine and bleomycin are useful in KS. Lymphomas may respond to cyclophosphamide or standard combination regimens.
3. *Antimicrobial chemotherapy*: treated early, PCP often responds to high dose co-trimoxazole. Oral co-trimoxazole or inhaled pentamidine are used for primary or secondary prophylaxis. CMV infections are treated with foscarnet or ganciclovir. Herpes virus infections usually respond to aciclovir. Superficial mycoses respond to topical nystatin or miconazole, but for deep infections, e.g. cryptococcosis or invasive candidosis, amphotericin B (usually lipid complexed) and/or fluconazole or itraconazole are used. Therapy for cerebral toxoplasmosis and parasitic gut disease, e.g. cryptosporidiosis, remains unsatisfactory. Bacterial infections are treated with standard antibiotics. MAC infections may respond to high dose clarithromycin or azithromycin but are often resistant even to combinations of anti-mycobacterial therapy.

Prevention

No vaccines are currently available. Prevention consists of risk reduction and education. Blood, blood products and donor organs are carefully screened, casual sexual encounters are discouraged and condom use is recommended. IV drug misusers should join withdrawal programmes or substitute oral methadone. Free sterile injection equipment and condoms should be available. Public awareness of risk must be encouraged, notably regarding casual unprotected heterosexual and homosexual male intercourse. HIV infection is either reportable or statutorily notifiable (in strict confidence), as is developed AIDS, in most countries of the world.

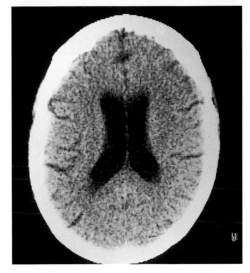

Fig. 168 Encephalopathy/cerebral atrophy in HIV infection.

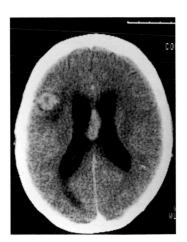

Fig. 169 Toxoplasma encephalitis: ring lesion on CT scan.

Index

124